DISEASE
Second Edition

Kenneth L. Jones
Louis W. Shainberg
Curtis O. Byer

Mt. San Antonio College

CANFIELD PRESS
San Francisco
A Department of Harper & Row, Publishers, Inc.

DISEASE, Second Edition

Copyright © 1975 by Kenneth L. Jones, Louis W. Shainberg, and Curtis O. Byer

Library of Congress Cataloging in Publication Data

Jones, Kenneth Lamar, 1931–
  Disease.

  First ed. published in 1970 under title: Communicable and noncommunicable diseases.
  Bibliography
  Includes index.
  1. Communicable diseases.   2. Diseases—Causes and
theories of causation.   I. Shainberg, Louis W., joint
author.   II. Byer, Curtis O., joint author.
III. Title. [DNLM: 1. Communicable diseases—Popular
works.   2. Medicine—Popular works. WB130 J77c]
RC113.J65   1975   616.07   75-1404
ISBN 0-06-384301-3

Interior and cover design by Penny Faron

76 77   10 9 8 7 6 5 4 3 2

PREFACE

Disease has afflicted people throughout history and will be with us for some time to come. Although the communicable diseases present less of a public health hazard than they once did, much of our population continues to suffer from them. The noncommunicable diseases have now become the leading causes of death in the United States. Today many diseases are entirely preventable by immunization, some are still only controllable, and others continue to elude science completely.

Ironically, the great strides which science has made in preventive medicine have resulted in a general lack of concern and responsibility on the part of the individual. Informed and motivated individuals can greatly reduce their own chances of being victims of diseases which cause disability or death. The purpose of this book is to help provide the information and motivation to prevent diseases or to minimize their damaging effects if they occur.

K. L. J.
L. W. S.
C. O. B.

CONTENTS

Chapter 1
PRINCIPLES OF COMMUNICABLE DISEASES

Communicable diseases are diseases that can be transmitted from one person or animal to another. Such diseases are also called *infectious* and *contagious*. One characteristic common to all communicable diseases is that they are caused by the parasitism of some living organism in man. These organisms are commonly called "germs" or, more properly, *pathogens*. A pathogen is any disease-producing organism (living thing) or material. Infectious diseases are all diseases caused by organisms; communicable diseases are those infectious diseases that can be transmitted.

Pathogens

Every communicable or infectious disease that causes illness in humans is the result of parasitism by some living organism. These disease-producing organisms are pathogens (commonly called "germs"). Most, although not all, pathogens are microscopic in size and are, therefore, sometimes referred to as *microbes* or *microorganisms*. Only a small percentage of known microorganisms are human pathogens, many others are highly beneficial to humans, and still others produce disease in plants and animals other than humans.

A disease is usually the result of some aspect of a pathogen's life processes, rather than of its mere presence. A healthy person harbors many microorganisms. Some are beneficial, such as the intestinal bacteria that produce vitamins. Others are potential pathogens, capable of producing disease under certain conditions. Still others have been shown to be neither beneficial nor harmful.

Biologists have classified all living things into groups that have common basic characteristics. Groups that include important pathogens are summarized in Table 1.1, which is arranged in order from the smallest to the largest.

TABLE 1.1   Groups of Organisms Containing Important Pathogens

Group	Brief Description	Size Range
Viruses	Subcellular, semiliving particles; similar to genes	10–250 nanometers (millimicrons)[a]
Bacteria	Single-celled, plantlike organisms	1–10 micrometers (microns)[a]
Protozoa	Single-celled animals	2–250 micrometers
Fungi	Single-celled or multicellular plantlike organisms, including molds, mushrooms, and yeasts	From a few micrometers to several inches
Parasitic worms	Multicellular animals; flat or round	From 1/32 inch to 20 or 30 feet

[a] One micrometer (formerly the micron) is 0.000039 inch; one nanometer (formerly the millimicron) is 0.000000039 inch. A micrometer is a millionth of a meter and a nanometer is a billionth of a meter.

Viruses

Viruses (Figure 1.1) are the smallest known pathogens. Viruses are the causative agents for such troublesome ailments as the common cold and influenza, as well as for less prevalent diseases such as poliomyelitis, rabies, and yellow fever. Viruses are not visible with even the most powerful light microscope, but they can be studied with an electron microscope.

Virus particles lack the more complex cellular structure that is characteristic of most plants and animals. A typical virus particle essentially consists of a central core of genetic material, either ribonucleic acid (RNA) or deoxyribonucleic acid (DNA), enclosed within a protein coating.

Viruses lie at the borderline between living and nonliving matter. They are incapable of unassisted self-reproduction, growth, production of energy, and other vital processes of more sophisticated life forms. Viruses must live and reproduce *within* the living cell of some

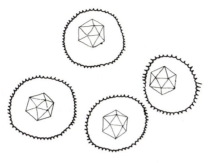

Figure 1.1 *A typical virus, as enlarged by an electron microscope. Note the angular shape characteristic of many kinds of viruses.*

host organism; thus they are all intracellular parasites. When a virus particle invades a suitable host cell, the genetic material of the virus is believed to act as a "gene" which assumes control of the cell and "tricks" the cell into manufacturing more virus material. The normal functioning of the cell is thereby disrupted, often with serious consequences. Cells may be only temporarily affected, producing such minor afflictions as colds, or they may be permanently damaged, producing such serious diseases as polio (and possibly cancer).

Certain viruses, such as herpes simplex, are known for their ability to lie dormant (*latent* infection) for long periods of time.

Bacteria

Bacteria are microscopic single-celled plantlike organisms. Although they are hundreds of times larger than viruses, they are barely visible with light microscopes of one-thousand-power magnification.

It is fortunate that most bacteria are not pathogenic to man because bacteria are almost everywhere. They are abundant in the air, in most city water supplies, in pasteurized milk, and in soil. The human body harbors many harmless bacteria. Millions are present in the mouth and intestines and on the skin and hair. Some of these normally harmless bacteria may cause severe infections under certain conditions, such as when a person is weakened through malnutrition or another disease.

Bacteria cause diseases by releasing *toxins* (poisons) and *enzymes* (substances having the ability to produce chemical changes). These toxins and enzymes cause the death and destruction of human body cells. In some infections the toxins and enzymes have only a localized effect, destroying the tissues near the infection. The toxins of other bacteria may be carried by the blood to cause damage throughout the body. Some bacteria release enzymes that destroy the red blood cells.

There are two basic types of toxins, *exotoxins* and *endotoxins*. Exotoxins are released from living bacteria, while endotoxins are released following the death of the bacteria. Of the two, the exotoxins are much more toxic and include the toxins of tetanus and botulism, some of the most poisonous substances known to man. On the other hand, it is often possible to produce immunization against exotoxins, but seldom against endotoxins.

TYPES OF BACTERIA

The hundreds of different kinds of bacteria can be organized into three groups on the basis of their shape. This surface appearance, however, gives little indication of their ability to cause disease. Even when examined under the best microscope, a dangerous type of bacterium might look exactly like a harmless type. Nevertheless, recognition of the shape of the bacteria found in a particular disease or infection is often useful in diagnoses. The three basic shapes are:

1. *Spheres.* The spherical bacteria are called *cocci* (the singular form is *coccus*). Figure 1.2 shows several important forms of cocci.

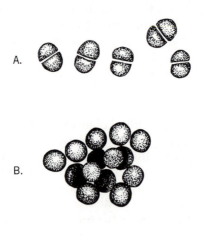

A.

B.

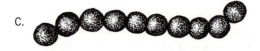

C.

Figure 1.2 *Spherical bacteria (cocci). (A) Diplococci, different species of which cause gonorrhea, pneumonia, and meningitis; (B) staphylococci, which cause boils and other infections; (C) streptococci, forms of which cause strep throat, rheumatic fever, scarlet fever, and other infections.*

2. *Rods*. The rod-shaped bacteria are called *bacilli* (the singular form is *bacillus*). Figure 1.3 shows some typical bacilli.

3. *Spirals*. The spiral or corkscrew-shaped bacteria are called *spirilla* (the singular form is *spirillum*) or *spirochetes*. Figure 1.4 illustrates some common types of spirilla.

Fungi

Fungi (singular *fungus*) are primitive plants. Familiar fungi are mushrooms, toadstools, yeasts, and the molds that grow on bread, cheese, and other foods. The fungus that causes the disease commonly called athlete's foot is shown in Figure 1.5. Like most fungi, it consists of threadlike strands and reproduces by forming numerous spores.

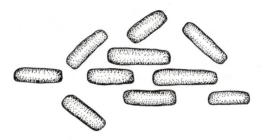

Figure 1.3 *Rod-shaped bacteria (bacilli). Various bacilli are responsible for tuberculosis, tetanus, and other diseases.*

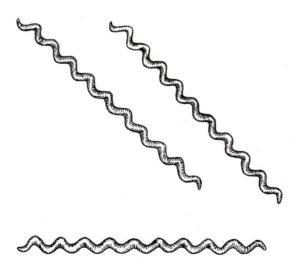

Figure 1.4 *Spiral bacteria (spirilla or spirochetes). An important disease caused by a spirochete is syphilis.*

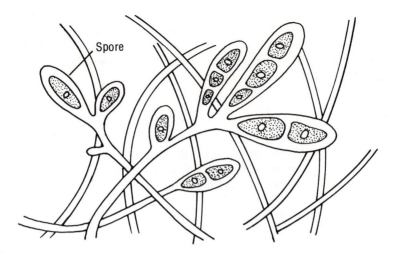

Figure 1.5 *A typical fungus. This fungus is the cause of athlete's foot and similar skin infections. Note the spores by which fungi reproduce.*

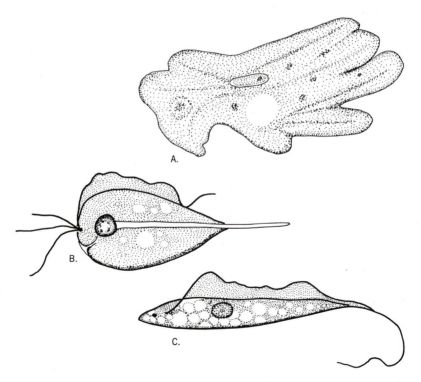

Figure 1.6 *Some typical protozoa (single-celled animals). (A) Ameba; (B) trichomonad; (C) typanosome.*

When these spores find their way to an appropriate part of the body, they produce a new growth of fungus, resulting in disease. Fungi most commonly cause diseases of the skin, hair, nails, and lungs of man, although several fungus diseases occur in other parts of the body. Some diseases caused by fungi include ringworm, coccidioidomycosis (valley fever), and histoplasmosis.

Protozoa

Protozoa (Figure 1.6) are microscopic animals. The entire body of each animal consists of just one cell. The smallest protozoa are no larger than bacteria; the largest are barely visible to the naked eye.

Protozoan diseases of man are most prevalent in tropical areas and areas with poor sanitation. Some important protozoan diseases are malaria, amebic dysentery, and African sleeping sickness. One protozoan, *Trichomonas*, causes a vaginal infection common among women in the United States.

Parasitic Worms

The largest pathogens are the *parasitic worms*. Their size varies from a fraction of an inch to 60 feet long. The two basic types of worms are flatworms (Figure 1.7) and roundworms (Figure 1.8).

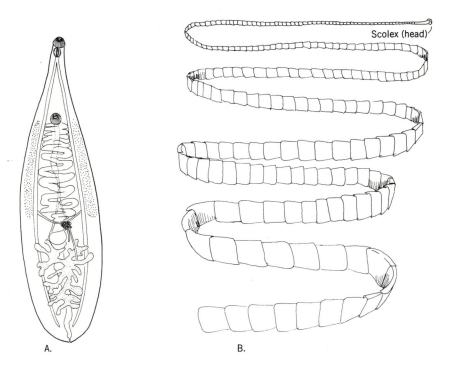

A.   B.

Figure 1.7 *Parasitic flatworms. (A) Fluke; (B) tapeworm.*

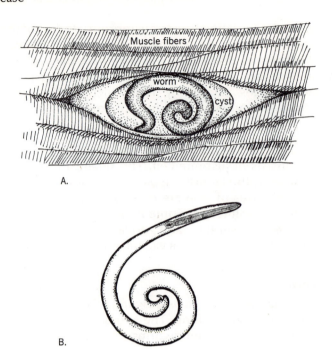

Figure 1.8 *Parasitic roundworms. (A) Trichinella worm in muscle (trichinosis disease); (B) pinworm.*

Stages of Communicable Disease

Most communicable diseases progress through several definite stages. These stages are discussed in the following sections and shown in Figure 1.9.

Transmission and Infection

For every disease there is some *reservoir of infection*. The reservoir may be humans, animals, insects, soil—wherever the pathogen normally lives and multiplies. The reservoir is the principle source of the pathogen, from which it can be transmitted to susceptible persons. For many diseases, such as gonorrhea and typhoid fever, symptomless human carriers are the principle reservoirs of infection.

Transmission is any mechanism by which a pathogen is carried from its reservoir to a susceptible person. Some of the more common methods of transmission include:

1. *Direct contact,* such as touching, kissing, or sexual contact
2. *Indirect contact,* through contaminated objects such as eating utensils, toys, or clothing

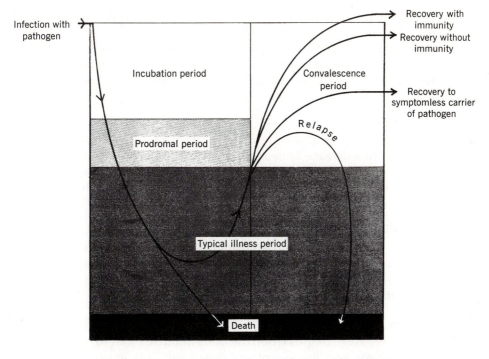

Figure 1.9 *The stages of a communicable disease from infection to death or recovery.*

3. *Airborne particles,* such as when pathogens discharged from the nose or mouth or originating from contaminated soil or objects float in the air as dust particles
4. *Contaminated food, milk, or water.*
5. *Insects or other arthropod vectors,* such as infected mosquitoes which transmit malaria

Infection occurs when the pathogen enters the body and begins to multiply or develop. Not every exposure to a pathogen results in infection. In fact, most of us are in daily contact with many different pathogens, but our body defenses prevent them from establishing infection.

Incubation Period

Once a communicable disease has been caught, it progresses through an *incubation period,* the interval between the time of infection and the appearance of the first symptoms of a disease. During this time, the pathogen multiplies until it is abundant enough to overcome body defenses and produce its disease.

The incubation period may be as short as a few hours or as long as several years, depending on the disease. Most diseases have an incubation period of a few days to a few weeks. Generally, diseases are not contagious during the early part of the incubation period, but they do become highly contagious at the end of the period, just before the symptoms appear.

Prodromal Period

The *prodromal period* is the time during which vague, non-specific symptoms of a disease appear. This period lasts from a few hours to several days and is characterized by fever, headache, and various aches and pains. Many diseases are highly contagious during this period.

Typical Illness Stage

After the prodromal period a group of specific symptoms appears. The term *syndrome* is often used to indicate a group of symptoms characteristic of a given disease. In this *typical illness stage,* a recognizable disease is present.

Recovery Stage

The *recovery stage* begins when the body defenses start to overpower the pathogens and the symptoms disappear. It is important to remember that the pathogens are still present in the body during the recovery or *convalescence* stage. If a convalescent person resumes full activity too soon, his body defenses may be weakened, and he may have a *relapse* (return of symptoms of the disease).

Symptomless Human Carriers of Disease

Symptomless human carriers are either people who have never shown symptoms of some disease or people who have recovered from the disease but continue to carry the pathogen and transmit it to others. For example, in at least 10–20 percent of infected males and 80–90 percent of infected females, gonorrhea is symptomless. Recent studies have shown that, following recovery from infectious mononucleosis, some people continue to discharge the virus for up to 16 months. Symptomless carriers of typhoid fever may discharge the bacterium for many years. The most famous typhoid carrier was Mary Mallon, better known as "Typhoid Mary." She was a cook, and wherever she worked outbreaks of typhoid fever would follow. After at least 10 outbreaks, she was confined to a special home and was not allowed to leave or to cook for any of her visitors. For some diseases, symptomless carriers are the most important reservoirs of pathogens.

Protection Against Communicable Diseases

Not too many years ago, communicable diseases were the major cause of death in the United States. (The average life span then was about 25 years less than it is today.) Now the deaths resulting from these diseases have been greatly reduced in the United States and in many other countries. But this reduction does not mean that we can forget about the diseases. The germs are still around us. Only by continuing to use all the known protective measures can we continue to control communicable diseases. Some of the important defenses against communicable diseases are discussed under five categories: public health measures, personal prevention, natural body defenses, immunization, and drugs.

Public Health Measures

Many types of protection against disease are impossible or extremely difficult for an individual to carry out. The responsibility for these types of protection, therefore, has been assumed by federal, state, county, or city agencies and by specially formed districts. These public health activities include:

1. Food and meat inspection
2. Dairy inspection and the testing of cows and milk
3. Restaurant inspection
4. Water testing
5. Sewage disposal
6. Rodent control
7. Mosquito and fly control
8. Discovery and treatment of carriers of diseases
9. Immunization for prevention of diseases

Personal Prevention

All too often, disease and its consequences seem unimportant until it is too late for even the most advanced medical science to be of help. While some methods of disease prevention are public health concerns, the individual is responsible for basic measures to prevent disease and to detect and treat it early.

Many communicable diseases can be prevented through immunization at the correct times, followed by boosters when necessary. It is extremely important that children receive adequate immunization, not only for their own protection but for that of the community as well. But for other important communicable diseases, for which effective immunizations are yet to be developed, including both syphilis and gonorrhea, prompt treatment is needed to prevent infecting others.

A periodic physical examination is essential to maintain health. A physician can detect many diseases even before visible symptoms occur, and successful treatment often depends upon early detection. Even cancer victims have a good chance of recovery if treatment is early enough. Routine testing can also detect infectious diseases like tuberculosis, or serious metabolic disorders like diabetes. During a physical many serious heart problems can be found which, if not treated, may lead to an early death.

Everyone should learn the danger signals of cancer and heart diseases. If any of them appear, a physician should be consulted immediately. A delay of only a few weeks in treatment may drastically reduce the chances for recovery.

The principles of nutrition should be learned and followed. Without the proper nutrients—proteins, carbohydrates, fatty acids, vitamins, and minerals—the body cannot maintain its defenses against disease. Excessive weight gains should be avoided, as obesity may be a contributive factor in many diseases. Also, sudden weight losses should be checked out by a physician as they may indicate serious problems, such as diabetes or tuberculosis. Exercise is equally important in maintaining health, especially of the heart and blood vessels.

When a family has reason to suspect transmission of a genetic disease, genetic counseling is available and should be sought out. This simple measure can prevent what might prove to be a tragedy for parents and child as well.

While the cost of medical care often seems prohibitive, disease prevention always proves less expensive than treatment. Many immunizations and diagnostic tests may be obtained at public health centers at minimal rates. If possible, every individual should arrange to be covered by a good-quality, high-limit, major medical insurance policy.

Natural Body Defenses

The human body has a great ability to resist disease. We are constantly being exposed to germs. Most of the time we completely resist these germs, and no infection occurs. When infection does take place, recovery is often possible through the body's own unassisted defenses. Some of these natural defenses are:

1. *Skin and mucous membranes.* The unbroken skin or mucous membrane keeps out most pathogens, even though a few can penetrate healthy skin.

2. *Tears.* Tears, constantly flowing over the surface of the eyes,

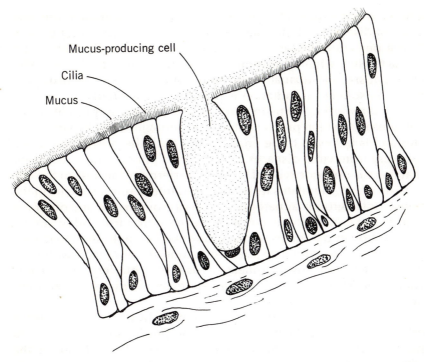

Mucus-producing cell

Cilia

Mucus

Figure 1.10 *Ciliated epithelium. Such cells form the lining of the ducts of the respiratory system. The cilia, through wavelike movement, carry foreign matter from the lungs.*

contain an enzyme *(lysozyme)* that destroys some bacteria. Without this enzyme, the eyes would have many more infections than they do.

3. *Cilia and mucus lining the respiratory system.* The ducts of the respiratory system have an inner lining of millions of *cilia* (Figure 1.10), microscopic hairs that pick up inhaled bacteria, dust, and foreign matter on a thin layer of mucus. The cilia wave in such a manner that the mucus and foreign matter is carried up to the throat and swallowed. This action helps keep the lungs free of infection. In the heavy smoker these cilia may completely disappear. The smoker then must cough frequently to clear foreign matter from the lungs. Years of coughing may contribute to emphysema, a serious condition in which the air sacs of the lungs break down (see Chapter 4).

4. *White blood cells.* There are five principal types of white blood cells or *leukocytes* (see Figure 5.2). Certain of these leukocytes are able to engulf bacteria and digest them, a process called *phagocytosis.* Other leukocytes produce antibodies, discussed in paragraph 6 below. The total number of the white blood cells present

and the number of each type (the "count") is important in the diagnosis of disease. The normal total count varies from about 6,000 to 10,000 per cubic millimeter of blood. An abnormally high count, characteristic when infection is present in the body, is called *leukocytosis*; an unusually low count, often the result of drug reactions, poisoning, or radiation exposure, is called *leukopenia*.

5. *Interferon*. Virus-infected cells release a protein called "*interferon*," which protects other cells from invasion by virus particles and is believed to be important in both the prevention of and recovery from virus diseases. Interferon is not specific in the sense that there is only one type of human interferon regardless of the type of virus which stimulates its production. Interferon *is* specific in that human interferon is apparently different from that of any other animal; thus it is of no value to isolate the interferon from other animals for injection into humans. A promising clinical application to disease prevention is to stimulate the production of interferon within the body by introducing harmless viruses or interferon-stimulating chemicals. This process is still in the experimental stage and may never be a practical reality.

6. *Antibodies*. The invasion of the body by pathogens or certain other foreign substances stimulates the production of *antibodies*, proteins which destroy the foreign substances. The substances that stimulate the production of antibodies are called *antigens*. A specific antibody usually destroys only the type of antigen that caused the production of the antibody. Antibodies are the basis of *immunity*. A person who is *immune* to a disease produces antibodies against that disease. Antibodies are one of the most important natural defenses against disease; they are the basis for the protection given by immunization.

Immunization

Through *immunization*, a person can develop immunity to many important diseases without having to suffer from them. There are two basic methods of immunization. *Active immunity* is obtained by injecting or otherwise exposing a person to an antigen, which causes the person to produce his own antibodies. The resulting immunity is usually long-lasting; that is, it is effective for several years or even for a lifetime. *Passive immunity* is obtained by injecting a person with antibodies extracted from the blood of an animal or from another person. Passive immunity is instantaneous, but of short duration. The injected antibodies break down in a few weeks without stimulating the person to produce antibodies of his own. Only his exposure to antigens can give him long-term protection.

A special type of passive immunity is *congenital immunity*. During pregnancy, antibodies pass across the placenta from the blood of the mother into the blood of the child. These antibodies give the newborn child immunity against many common diseases. But since this is passive immunity, it lasts only for several months. The proper protection of an infant involves a series of injections given at regular intervals during the first few years of life, starting at about age 2 months. It is the responsibility of parents to see that their child receives these immunizations or "shots." Every child born in the United States should be immunized against seven diseases: diphtheria, tetanus, whooping cough, polio, measles, German measles, and mumps. It should be remembered that continued protection against diphtheria and tetanus requires booster immunizations every ten years throughout adult life.

Immunizations against several other common diseases are still being developed and may eventually become part of the standard immunization series. In addition, immunizations against many other diseases, for example, smallpox, cholera, plague, yellow fever, and typhoid fever, are already available for use in special cases, such as before travel into foreign countries.

Drugs

The use of drugs to treat diseases is called *chemotherapy*. In general, the drugs developed so far have had the greatest success against bacterial diseases, moderate success against protozoan and fungal diseases and parasitic worms, and little or no effect on the viral diseases. A few antiviral drugs have been developed, however, and there is good probability that others will come eventually.

The discovery of *sulfa drugs* (sulfonamides) in 1935 was the first major step toward the control of bacterial infection. These drugs are chemically produced and are usually taken by mouth. They prevent the multiplication of bacteria by chemically mimicking a vitamin (para-aminobenzoic acid) needed by bacteria but not by man. Important bacterial enzyme systems are blocked. Since the bacteria are not killed, just inhibited, it is important that the drug be taken for an adequate time to allow the body defenses, such as white blood cells and antibodies, to destroy the bacteria. Sulfa drugs are excreted in the urine, so are ideal for certain urinary infections. When taking sulfa drugs, it is important to drink plenty of fluids; if water intake is too low, the drugs may crystalize in the tubules of the kidneys, causing severe kidney damage.

Antibiotics are substances that are produced in soil-inhabiting microorganisms in order to inhibit the growth of competing soil organisms. Antibiotics are made for drug use by growing the organisms that produce them in large vats of liquid. From this liquid, antibiotics are extracted and then purified. Most antibiotics are given by injection, but some are effective if taken by mouth.

Antibiotics are generally effective only against bacteria; they have no effect on viruses. Antibiotics cannot cure a cold, influenza, measles, mumps, or other viral disease.

Several problems have arisen as the result of intensive antibiotic use. One problem has been the development of drug resistance among many kinds of bacteria, rendering them difficult or impossible to control with antibiotics. To minimize the development of such resistant bacteria, indiscriminate use of antibiotics should be avoided. If an antibiotic must be used, the physician's instructions should be followed explicitly. Another problem has been the development of allergies in patients with repeated antibiotic use. In their more severe form, these allergies may be fatal (anaphylactic shock). It is important that the physician be told of any drug reaction, no matter how slight. Even the appearance of a mild rash may be evidence that a drug allergy is developing which, with further exposure to the same drug, could be fatal.

When taking medications, the following precautions should be observed:

1. *Follow instructions exactly.* To be effective, drugs must be present in the blood at adequate levels for adequate periods of time. Haphazard taking of medication (e.g., skipping pills and "doubling up" later) cannot achieve this result. The full course of prescribed treatment should always be taken. Never stop taking a medication just because the outward symptoms of an infection have disappeared—there are often live pathogens remaining in the body which the remaining medication may be necessary to help control.

2. *Use a drug only for the illness for which it was prescribed.* Do not keep left over drugs for future use. The same drug might not be at all appropriate for a future illness. Also, many drugs break down in storage and become worthless or even harmful.

3. *Never borrow or lend prescriptions.* Different diseases may have similar symptoms, and a borrowed prescription may be dangerous. In some cases it is even illegal to possess a prescription drug without having a prescription.

4. *Keep all drugs out of the reach of children, in a locked cabinet.* Do not underestimate the ability of children to climb and reach medications stored in high places.

5. *Avoid unnecessary use of antibiotics.* Never press a physician to prescribe an antibiotic for a virus condition, for which it can do no good at all.

The Host–Parasite Relationship: A Dynamic Interaction

Infectious disease can be best understood if seen as a dynamic conflict between the host (person) and the parasite (pathogen). Every day of his life, a person is exposed to infectious agents which, given the opportunity, can result in illness or even death. These pathogens need to establish parasitism on the person in order to survive. The survival of the person, in turn, depends upon the body defenses overcoming the pathogens. Fortunately, the body defenses are usually strong enough to overcome most "everyday" pathogens. Disease usually results only when an unusually virulent pathogen is encountered or when the strength of the body defenses is reduced by such factors as injury, poor nutrition, or emotional stress.

Disease and health can be visualized as a balance with body defenses on one side and the virulence and number of pathogens on the other. When someone is getting sick the balance is tipped in favor of the pathogen. When someone is getting well or maintaining good health the balance is tipped in favor of the body defenses.

The usual role of drugs in treating infections is not to wipe out the pathogens unaided, but to help tip the balance in the dynamic host–parasite relationship to favor the host.

Stress and Disease

Hans Selye, the noted Canadian physiologist, has made important contributions to our understanding of the dynamics of disease. According to Selye, *stress,* in its most general sense, is a group of changes within a living system (such as a person) resulting from the imposition on the system of any harmful external force, or *stressor.* Some stressors are emotional conflict, fear, fatigue, physical injury, poor nutrition, disease pathogens, poison, and radiation.

Selye describes the *general adaptation syndrome,** a group of physical reactions elicited by any of these stressors. He emphasizes that regardless of the nature of the stressor, the reaction is the same. The general adaptation syndrome includes three successive stages. The first is the *alarm reaction,* consisting of the immediate mobilization of the body's defense mechanisms. If the stress continues for some time, however, the person enters the second stage, called *resistance to stress.* This is the stage of maximum ability to withstand the stressor. It may continue for days, weeks, or even months, depending on the vitality of the person and the amount of rest he is able to obtain during this period of maximum effort. Such endurance, however, puts a considerable strain on the body's resources. If the stress continues long enough, the third stage, *exhaustion,* may be reached, in which the person becomes progressively devitalized and his ability to resist the stress diminishes. He has exhausted his internal resources for dealing with continued stress. Every function of the body is weakened. If this stage continues long enough, death results.

*Selye, Hans, *The Stress of Life,* New York: McGraw-Hill, 1956.

A key concept in the general adaptation syndrome is that since all types of stressors produce the same reaction, exposure to any one type of stressor reduces our ability to defend ourselves against all other types of stressors. For example, prolonged emotional stress interferes with our ability to fight off infectious diseases; thus, we may become physically ill more readily while under a stage of emotional stress. Or, conversely, physical illness lowers our ability to resist emotional stresses. Thus, the health of the body and of the mind are interdependent.

Summary

I. Communicable Diseases

    A. Diseases that can be caught—infectious or contagious diseases

    B. Caused by the parasitism of some living organism

II. Pathogens—Disease-producing Organism or Materials

    A. Infection—invasion of body by pathogens

    B. Groups of organisms containing important pathogens:

        1. Viruses—intracellular parasites; cause disease such as rabies, polio, and yellow fever, as well as colds and influenza

        2. Bacteria—release toxins and enzymes:

            a. Spheres—cocci

            b. Rods—bacilli

            c. Spirals—spirilla, spirochetes

        3. Fungi—primitive plants; cause diseases of the skin, hair, nails and lungs

        4. Protozoa—one-celled animals; cause diseases such as malaria, amebic dysentery, and African sleeping sickness

        5. Parasitic worms—flatworms, roundworms

III. Stages of Communicable Disease

    A. Transmission—pathogen is carried from the source, enters body, through:

        1. Direct contact

        2. Indirect contact

        3. Airborne particles

        4. Contaminated food, milk, or water

        5. Insects or other arthropod vectors

    B. Infection—pathogen establishes itself in body

    C. Incubation period—interval between infection and appearance of first symptoms

D. Prodromal period—nonspecific symptoms appear, highly contagious stage

E. Typical illness stage—specific symptoms appear

F. Recovery stage—body defenses overpower pathogens

G. Symptomless carriers—important in transmission of many diseases

IV. Protection against Communicable Diseases

  A. Public health measures:

    1. Food, milk, and restaurant inspection

    2. Water testing and sewage disposal

    3. Rodent, mosquito, and fly control

    4. Discovery and treatment of carriers of disease

    5. Immunization

  B. Personal prevention

    1. Immunization

    2. Prompt treatment to prevent infecting others

    3. Periodic physical exams

    4. Know danger signals of cancer and heart diseases

    5. Proper nutrition and weight control

    6. Genetic counseling

    7. Good health insurance

  C. Natural body defenses

    1. Skin and mucous membranes—barriers to many pathogens

    2. Tears—contain enzyme (lysozyme) that destroys some bacteria

    3. Cilia of respiratory tract—sweep out pathogens and other foreign matter

    4. White blood cells—engulf bacteria (phagocytosis) and produce antibodies

    5. Interferon—produced by virus-infected cells to protect other cells from infection

    6. Antibodies—produced in response to the presence of antigens, destroy specific antigens

  D. Immunization—two basic methods:

    1. Active immunity

      a. Antigen enters body, stimulates production of antibodies

      b. Generally long-lasting

    2. Passive immunity

      a. Injection of antibodies provides instant immunity

    b. Has short duration of effectiveness

    c. Congenital immunity—antibodies are passed from pregnant woman to unborn child

  3. Every child should be immunized against:

    a. Diphtheria

    b. Tetanus

    c. Whooping cough

    d. Polio

    e. Measles

    f. German measles

    g. Mumps

E. Drugs—chemotherapy

  1. Sulfa drugs

    a. Inhibit but do not kill bacteria

    b. Ideal for urinary infections

    c. Patient should drink plenty of water

  2. Antibiotics

    a. Effective against many bacteria; no effect on viruses

    b. Many bacteria are becoming resistant

    c. Patient must be alert to development of allergy

  3. When taking medications:

    a. Follow instructions exactly

    b. Use a drug only for the illness for which it was prescribed

    c. Never borrow or lend prescriptions

    d. Keep all drugs out of reach of children, in a locked cabinet

    e. Avoid unnecessary use of antibiotics

V. The Host–Parasite Relationship: A Dynamic Interaction

  A. Every day a person is exposed to many pathogens

  B. Body defenses are usually strong enough to overcome "everyday" pathogens

  C. Disease results when:

    1. An unusually virulent pathogen is encountered

    2. Body defenses are weakened

  D. Role of drugs is to tip balance in host-parasite relationship to favor the host

VI. Stress and Disease

A. A variety of stressors—emotional conflict, fatigue, physical injury, poor nutrition, disease pathogens, and others—elicit the same body response, the general adaptation syndrome.

B. Three stages in this syndrome:

    1. Alarm reaction

    2. Resistance to stress

    3. Exhaustion—ability to resist stress diminishes

C. Exposure to any one stressor reduces ability to defend against others.

    1. Emotional stress reduces ability to fight infectious disease.

    2. Physical illness lowers ability to resist emotional stresses.

Questions for Review

1. What is a communicable disease? What causes a communicable disease?
2. Name and briefly describe the major disease-producing organisms.
3. What are the stages of a communicable disease?
4. What requirements are necessary for the first stage to occur?
5. What are the modes of transmission by which diseases may be spread?
6. The human body has a great ability to resist disease. Describe the natural defenses the body has to fight infection.
7. List some of the public health measures that provide protection against disease.
8. Compare active and passive immunity. What is congenital immunity?
9. What are the differences between sulfa drugs and antibiotics? Are they used for the same purposes? Explain.
10. The indiscriminate use of antibiotics may have two undesirable effects. What are they? What other precautions should a person observe while taking drugs?
11. What is meant by "host-parasite relationship: a dynamic interaction"?
12. What is a syndrome?
13. What is the general adaptation syndrome?
14. Describe the interrelationship between emotional health and infectious disease.

Chapter 2
SOME IMPORTANT COMMUNICABLE DISEASES

Certain shared characteristics enable several diseases to be considered together as the common diseases.

Common Diseases

The group of common diseases includes some often called "childhood diseases" because the greatest number of cases are in the age group of one to fifteen years. Since these diseases usually confer lifelong immunity, repeated infection is not common. It is not unusual, however, for a person to escape infection during childhood and then catch one of these diseases as an adult.

Several other diseases in this group, such as the common cold and influenza, are actually groups of many similar diseases, each caused by a slightly different strain of pathogen. There is only limited cross-immunity between the strains and a relatively short-term immunity to any one of them. Thus colds and influenza can be caught repeatedly.

Chickenpox

Chickenpox is a highly contagious disease that usually confers lifetime immunity. Most cases occur in children between the ages of two and eight years. This combination of traits makes it a childhood disease.

Chickenpox is caused by a virus called the *varicella* virus. The same virus, when contracted by adults who have not had chickenpox, sometimes causes an infection of the nervous system called *shingles* or *Herpes zoster* (characterized by painful inflammation of the skin).

The characteristic symptoms of chickenpox are a mild fever and typical lesions on the skin. The disease is probably contagious from the day before eruption of the lesions until about six days after their eruption. The virus is transmitted through direct or indirect contact with the discharge from the skin lesions or with the nose or throat discharges (breath, saliva, sputum, and mucus) of infected persons. These discharges may be airborne for short distances.

The incubation period is usually fourteen to sixteen days, and the length of the disease that follows is usually nine to fourteen days. Permanent aftereffects of chickenpox are very rare. No effective vaccine has yet been released for clinical use.

The Common Cold

The most widespread infectious disease in the United States today is the *common cold*. Colds cause more discomfort, inconvenience, and lost time from work and school than any other disease. Although the common cold itself is not a serious disease, very serious side effects, such as secondary bacterial infections, may result from the improper care of patients with colds. Unfortunately, the common cold is one of the least preventable communicable diseases.

Colds are caused by viruses. Over fifty different viruses cause symptoms of the common-cold type. The first symptoms usually include a scratchy throat, stuffy nose, tiredness, and feeling cold in a room at normal temperature. Other symptoms include sneezing, coughing, and watering eyes. A high fever is *not* a normal symptom of a cold. When a high fever accompanies cold symptoms, a dangerous secondary infection or a more serious disease may be present. For this reason a physician should be consulted.

There is no specific way to prevent the common cold. No effective immunization has yet been developed, possibly because so many different viruses can cause cold symptoms and because the body produces no long-term immunity after actually having had a cold. It is debatable whether exposure to cold temperatures causes colds by making the mucous membranes more susceptible to cold viruses. In any case, a virus must be present to cause the disease. Therefore the most important means of preventing colds is to avoid unnecessary contact with people who have a cold.

One of the many controversies in modern medicine concerns the value of vitamin C (ascorbic acid) as a preventative or cure for colds. Various studies have given a mixed picture of the value of vitamin C for this purpose; qualified authorities can be cited to support either side of the question.* In any case, it is important to have at least an adequate level of vitamin C in the diet to allow general good health and maintain the various disease resistance mechanisms. At the same time it seems advisable to avoid the extremely high vitamin C levels (several grams per day) recommended by some individuals, in light of possible kidney damage to people with impaired kidney function or inadequate fluid intake.

Even if all known precautions are taken, the average person has at least one cold a year. He may then find dozens of remedies recommended to him. Some of these are highly advertised nonprescription medicines; others are home remedies suggested by friends and relatives. Unfortunately, none of these treatments actually cures a cold. Even the newest nonprescription remedies offer at best only partial relief from symptoms, not a cure.

The best treatment for a cold remains the same as it has been for many years: *Stay in bed during the early stages.* The result of trying to fight a cold with continued activity is often a serious secondary bacterial infection, especially of the ears, sinuses, or respiratory tract. Such an infection may last for weeks. In fact, any cold symptoms lingering after five to seven days probably result from such bacterial infections. Although antibiotics are not effective against the actual virus stage of a cold, they may be useful in clearing up the secondary bacterial infections.

Influenza

True *influenza,* or "flu," is a virus infection of the respiratory tract. The symptoms, which appear very suddenly, include fever, chills, headache, muscular aches, and coughing. The patient is usually completely disabled. Many other types of viral, and even bacterial, infections are commonly, though incorrectly, called "flu."

Influenza often occurs in massive epidemics, with so many disabled at the same time that the functioning of the community is disrupted. An otherwise healthy person rarely dies of influenza, but the death rate always rises during epidemics. Influenza deaths occur mainly among elderly persons or those already weakened by some chronic disease. Death is usually the result of pneumonia caused by secondary bacterial infections.

Influenza is transmitted though viruses present in the discharges from the nose and mouth of infected persons. Many strains of influenza viruses are known, and they fall into three basic types: A, B, and C. The Asian influenza is caused by one of the type A viruses.

The best prevention against influenza is vaccination. Annual booster vaccinations are necessary. Although vaccination does not

Medical World News, September 21, 1973, p. 52.

give absolute protection against influenza, it definitely reduces one's chances of having the disease and is especially recommended for pregnant women, elderly persons, and persons performing important community services.

Some Diseases Entirely Preventable by Immunization

Poliomyelitis (Polio)

Poliomyelitis, commonly called "polio," is completely preventable by proper immunization. However, cases continue to occur in the United States among people who have had only partial immunization or none at all.

Polio is caused by three different types of viruses, which produce diseases of different severity. *Paralytic polio,* leading to permanent paralysis or death, occurs when a polio virus invades the central nervous system. Fortunately, only a small percentage of polio cases are the paralytic type. In most cases the infection centers around the digestive tract and causes no permanent damage.

Two types of polio vaccines have been used. The first type, developed by Jonas Salk, is a killed virus vaccine given by injection. The second vaccine, developed by Albert Sabin, consists of live, *attenuated* (weakened) polio virus and is taken by mouth. The main polio vaccine in use today is the *Sabin oral polio vaccine* (OPV). Its advantages over the Salk vaccine include the fact that it is easier to give (or take) and that it results in a longer-lasting immunity.

The oral polio vaccine is currently given in a mixed form containing all three types of weakened polio viruses. This mixture is called *trivalent OPV.* If it is taken four times during childhood, a lifetime immunity results. The timing of doses is variable, but a typical schedule would include vaccination at two, four, and fifteen months of age and again at four to five years of age.

Smallpox

Throughout history smallpox has been among the most dreaded diseases. Today, through massive worldwide immunization programs, we can look forward to the eradication of this disease. Its occurrence has been reduced to limited areas of Asia and Africa.

Smallpox is caused by a highly contagious virus. It is transmitted by direct or indirect contact with the lesions that form on the skin or with the nose and throat discharges of infected persons. The disease is contagious from the beginning of the earliest symptoms until the skin lesions are entirely healed. Today about 25 percent of all smallpox cases result in death.

The vaccine used against smallpox contained the live virus (called *vaccinia virus*) of cowpox, a skin disease of cattle. When the vaccine is scratched into the skin, a small localized case of cowpox results at the point of the vaccination. The cowpox virus is so similar to the smallpox virus that the antibodies produced against one are effective against the other. Thus this harmless case of cowpox results in immunity to smallpox. The immunity gained from a smallpox vaccination lasts about ten years.

Because of the success of the smallpox eradication program, the United States Public Health Service no longer recommends routine smallpox immunization except for travel into areas where smallpox may still exist. This has caused some concern among physicians, but in recent years in the United States there have been between six and ten deaths a year from smallpox vaccination whereas there has not been a case of smallpox for many years. Of course, as a large unimmunized population develops here, it will be critically important to guard against an infected person entering the country in the event the world eradication program is not totally successful.

Measles (Rubeola)

Measles is a much more serious disease than is commonly believed. Only a few years ago, measles was thought of as a minor childhood disease. Few people realized that one in every fifteen infected children would have serious side effects, ranging from ear infections (with a chance of permanent deafness) to brain inflammation (which sent thousands of children to mental institutions for the rest of their lives). One in every thousand children suffering from measles died as a result of its side effects.

The cause of measles is a virus called the *rubeola virus*. The early symptoms of measles are similar to a cold but also include *Koplik's spots*—small bluish-white spots surrounded by red circular areas occuring on the mucous membranes in the mouth. Later, the dark-red rash typical of the disease appears.

The virus is transmitted through contact with the discharges from the nose, mouth, and eyes of an infected person. It is highly contagious from the first appearance of cold-type symptoms until the disappearance of such symptoms.

Fortunately, there is no need for any child today to suffer the discomfort of measles and to take the chance of its serious permanent effects. Since 1963 highly effective immunizations against measles have been available. The vaccine in use today contains live, attenuated measles virus. It should be given (by injection) to every infant when he reaches one year of age or soon thereafter. The single injection gives an active immunity against measles which is believed to last for a lifetime. Some states require immunization before a child can register for school.

Diphtheria

The incidence of *diphtheria* has been reduced greatly through the immunization of children. It occurs today mainly among low-income families where children are likely to receive inadequate immunization.

Diphtheria is caused by a rod-shaped bacterium called *Corynebacterium diphtheriae*. This bacterium usually grows on the mucous membranes of the throat and nose and occasionally on the skin. A gray membranelike material appears over the infected surfaces.

Diphtheria bacteria release a toxin which, when carried by the blood, has serious destructive effects on many parts of the body. This toxin causes the degeneration and death of tissues. The heart muscle and the nervous system are particularly easily damaged.

The bacteria are present in the nose and throat discharges of infected people and their transmission to another person is very possible since they can survive for several days outside the human body.

The immunizing agent used against diphtheria is a *toxoid*—a toxin that has been chemically treated so that it is no longer dangerous, but is still able to stimulate the production of antibodies. Diphtheria toxoid normally is given in combination with the immunizing agents for whooping cough (pertussis) and tetanus. This triple vaccine is referred to as *DPT vaccine*. Older children and adults often receive a combined diphtheria and tetanus booster shot, referred to as an adult *TD booster*. These immunizations may be given according to the schedule shown in Table 2.1, although some variation in timing is possible.

Whooping Cough (Pertussis)

In the United States today, *whooping cough* occurs mainly among young children from low-income families where adequate immunization practices are not always followed.

Whooping cough is caused by a rod-shaped bacterium called *Bordetella pertussis*. The center of infection in whooping cough is the respiratory tract. This infection causes great quantities of mucus to be produced. This mucus stimulates violent coughing spells during which five to fifteen or more coughs occur in rapid succession with no time for a breath between them. After each series of coughs, there is a rapid intake of air which produces a crowing sound or "whoop." Whooping cough is dangerous to young children, especially those under six months of age. Without proper treatment, the death rate can reach 25 percent; even the best treatment does not eliminate the threat of death entirely.

TABLE 2.1   Typical Immunization Schedule

Age	Vaccine
2 months	DPT (diphtheria, whooping cough, tetanus) Trivalent OPV (oral polio vaccine containing types I, II, and III)
3 months	DPT
4 months	DPT Trivalent OPV
12 months	Measles vaccine (live virus)
12 months to puberty	German measles vaccine Mumps vaccine
15 months	DPT Trivalent OPV
Before school entrance	DPT Trivalent OPV
15 years	TD (adult type tetanus and diphtheria booster)
Over 15 years	TD boosters every 10 years for life

Source: Advisory Committee on Immunization Practices Recommendations, U.S. Department of Health, Education, and Welfare, Center for Disease Control, Weekly Morbidity and Mortality Report, Supplement for June 24, 1972, and other sources.
Notes: 1. Routine smallpox immunization is no longer recommended by U.S. Public Health Service.
2. Measles, German measles, and mumps vaccines may be combined into a single trivalent vaccine.
3. This schedule is recommended as a flexible guide which may be modified within limits to meet the needs of the individual patient or physician.

There is no congenital immunity against whooping cough. An infant may be infected any time after birth, and 70 percent of the fatal cases occur before the age of one year. Thus an infant needs the protection of immunization as soon as possible. Immunization methods normally follow the series of DPT injections outlined in Table 2.1.

Tetanus (Lockjaw)

Tetanus, commonly called "lockjaw," is caused by a toxin released by *Clostridium tetani,* a spore-forming, rod-shaped bacterium. This organism lives in the intestines of animals, and its spores are contained in their feces. These spores remain alive for years and can be found in almost any soil.

Tetanus infection occurs when these spores enter a wound, which may be either deep or superficial and on any part of the body. When a tetanus infection occurs, the toxin released by the bacteria is picked up by the blood and acts on the central nervous system. This toxin causes constant impulses to run through the affected nerves. The muscles controlled by these nerves then have constant contrac-

TABLE 2.2 Tetanus Immunization Following Injury

History of Tetanus Immunization (Doses)	Clean, Minor Wounds		All Other Wounds	
	Td[a]	TIG[a]	Td	TIG
Uncertain	Yes	No	Yes	Yes
0–1	Yes	No	Yes	Yes
2	Yes	No	Yes	No[b]
3 or more	No[c]	No	No[d]	No

Source: Center for Disease Control Weekly Morbidity and Mortality Report, Vol. 20, No. 43, 1971.

[a] Td is adult type tetanus and diphtheria booster vaccine. TIG is Tetanus Immune Globulin (Human), an injection containing tetanus antitoxin (antibodies) and conferring immediate, passive immunity against tetanus.

[b] Unless wound more than 24 hours old.

[c] Unless more than 10 years since last dose.

[d] Unless more than 5 years since last dose.

tions, called *tetanus*. The most common early symptom of tetanus is stiffness of the jaw muscles, from which the common name "lock-jaw" is derived. Other symptoms may include restlessness, irritability, and stiffness of other parts of the body. The muscles gradually become more rigid, until repeated convulsions begin. Death, which occurs in about 50 percent of all cases even with proper treatment, often is caused by the failure of the muscles used for breathing.

People of all ages are susceptible to tetanus, and its prevention is a lifelong responsibility. Active immunity is achieved through injection with tetanus toxoid. As indicated in Table 2.1, this immunization should begin with the DPT shots of infancy and continue throughout adult life, as the immunity obtained from this toxoid is effective for only about ten years.

The question, "Should I get a tetanus shot?" frequently arises following injuries. Table 2.2 may help answer such questions. Policies of individual physicians vary, and many physicians take a cautious approach, recommending a booster immunization if more than two years have elapsed since the most recent tetanus immunization.

Incidentally, while people associate rusty nails with tetanus, rust has nothing to do with the condition. The spores of tetanus could just as well be carried by a shiny nail, a piece of glass, or a sharp wooden stick or splinter.

German Measles (Rubella)

German measles is also called *rubella* or "three-day measles." Like chickenpox, this is a virus-caused childhood disease, one attack of which *may* confer lifelong immunity. The age group usually affected is that from two to fifteen years, although the disease is fairly common in adults, and repeated attacks in the same person are not rare.

Typical symptoms of German measles include a mild rash, slight fever, and swelling of lymph glands in the neck. These symptoms usually appear from fourteen to twenty-one days after exposure and last for only one to four days. Transmission comes through contact with the nose or throat discharges of infected persons. The disease is contagious from one week before the rash appears until the rash disappears.

Permanent effects of German measles are rare except for damage to the unborn child when a woman is infected during the first six months of pregnancy. The chance of damage in such cases is very high during the first months of pregnancy and tapers off gradually through the sixth month. Typical types of resulting congenital damage are cataracts, deafness, heart defects, mental retardation, prematurity, and microcephaly (smallness of the head).

German measles is prevented by a highly effective vaccine that should be given during childhood. This vaccine must not be given to a pregnant woman or one who might become pregnant within two months of the shot, as the live virus of the vaccine may attack the unborn child.

Mumps

Mumps is another virus-caused disease. It most often occurs in childhood and usually leaves lifetime immunity. The common age of infection is from two to fourteen years.

The mumps virus is transmitted through direct or indirect contact with the nose or throat of an infected person. The symptoms, which usually appear sixteen to twenty days after exposure, include fever and a swelling and tenderness of the salivary glands. These symptoms last from four to ten days. The contagious period is from seven days before swelling appears until the swelling disappears.

Permanent effects are rare when cases occur before puberty. In males over fifteen years of age, however, there is about a 25-percent chance that one testis (rarely both) may be infected and degenerate. Infection of the ovaries of mature females is much less common, but can happen.

An effective, live-virus vaccine against mumps is available. It should be administered to all children over one year of age and to any adult who has never had mumps.

Some Other Important Diseases

Tuberculosis (TB)

During much of the history of the United States, *tuberculosis* reigned as the number one cause of death. Since the development of modern drug therapy, however, tuberculosis has become a fairly minor cause of death. Nevertheless, it remains an important disabling disease in this country and a major cause of death in many other countries.

Tuberculosis is caused by a rod-shaped bacterium called *Mycobacterium tuberculosis.* An important characteristic of this organism is its ability to remain alive for long periods of time outside the human body. It also has a high level of resistance to such forces as heat, drying, and many disinfectants.

Although the lungs are most commonly infected, any part of the body can be infected with tuberculosis. The main source of infection is bacteria that are contained in the respiratory discharges of infected persons and released in coughing, sneezing, or talking. Dried droplets of such discharges may be suspended in the air as dust particles. Tuberculosis infection most commonly occurs when such particles are inhaled into the lungs. Occasionally infections occur in those who drink raw milk from cows infected with the disease.

When the lungs are infected, the disease may proceed in one of several different ways. In rare cases, the infection spreads rapidly through the lungs, causing much destruction of tissue and the swift death of the person. More commonly, the infection spreads very slowly through the lungs and, if not treated, leads to death in several years. The bodies of many people are able to stop the spread of tuberculosis by walling off the infected area with a layer of special cells. This produces a nodule called a *tubercle.* The bacteria inside this tubercle may remain inactive but alive for several years. The ability to resist tuberculosis in this way depends upon general good health, including good nutrition. After several years of inactivity, a case of tuberculosis may become active if the physical condition of the person is weakened through malnutrition, excess fatigue, or another disease.

The main way to prevent tuberculosis is to avoid contact with known or suspected active cases and to avoid places frequented by such people. Tuberculosis is very common among derelicts and vagrants. Any place frequented by such people is likely to be contaminated with the bacteria of tuberculosis. Routine testing of cows and pasteurization of milk are also important in eliminating milk-borne tuberculosis.

Since tuberculosis is still very much present in the United States, the chances of exposure to the disease are not remote. It is very important, therefore, for every person to be periodically checked for the presence of tuberculosis. There are two methods of screening in common use today. Each has definite advantages and disadvantages. These two methods are chest X rays and skin tests.

Chest X rays are valuable for detecting tuberculosis and other lung disorders. They are the easiest way to test large numbers of people. They cannot, however, definitely distinguish tuberculosis from certain other disorders; nor can they distinguish active from inactive tuberculosis. Naturally, they cannot detect tuberculosis in any other part of the body.

In skin testing, an extract of killed tuberculosis bacteria, called *tuberculin,* is injected or scratched into the skin. If the person has some degree of or *has ever had* tuberculosis, redness will appear at the point of the injection. Like chest X rays, skin tests cannot distinguish active from inactive cases. But unlike chest X rays, skin tests detect tuberculosis occurring *anywhere in the body.*

If both the skin test and X ray are positive, the confirming test for active tuberculosis is (1) the presence of tuberculosis bacteria in the sputum or elsewhere in the body or (2) advancement in the degree of involvement as shown in the X ray.

A vaccine against tuberculosis is used in several other countries, but is seldom used in the United States because of its interference with skin tests for tuberculosis. Anyone who has had the vaccine will have a positive skin test. This vaccine (BCG) is sometimes used, however, for high-risk persons, such as nurses or children in contact with active cases of tuberculosis.

Though the treatment of tuberculosis has been greatly improved, it remains a slow process. People with active cases should be temporarily hospitalized to prevent the infection of family and other contacts. Usually the patient becomes noninfective within a few weeks after treatment begins; he can then resume normal contacts without endangering others. A complete cure, however, will take much longer.

Viral Hepatitis

"Hepatitis" is the general term applied to infection or inflammation of the liver. The term "jaundice" is sometimes associated with hepatitis. Jaundice is not a specific disease, but is, however, an important symptom of hepatitis. It is a yellowing of the skin, indicating an impairment of liver function. The liver is not removing enough bile pigment from the blood, so this pigment is deposited in the skin.

Viral liver infections are a major health problem today. While the exact number of viruses attacking the liver is unknown, most authorities cite two major types of viral hepatitis—infectious hepatitis and serum hepatitis. Each disease is believed to be caused by a different virus. Infectious hepatitis is caused by virus A, while serum hepatitis is the result of virus B, also called the Australia or serum hepatitis (SH) antigen. Either may range in severity from very mild to very serious, may require a long period of convalescence, and may occasionally cause death. Serum hepatitis is usually the more severe of the two. Their characteristics are compared in Table 2.3.

TABLE 2.3   Viral Infections of the Liver

Pathogen	Infectious Hepatitis Virus A	Serum Hepatitis Virus B
People usually affected	More common in children and young adults	More common in adults than children
Sources of virus	Blood, feces, and nose and throat discharges of infected persons	Blood of infected persons
Transmission	Direct contact, airborne spread, contaminated food or water, blood or blood products, contaminated injection needles and syringes, tattoo needles	Blood or blood products, contaminated injection needles and syringes, tattoo needles
Incubation period	10–50 days, commonly about 30–35 days	50–180 days, commonly 80–100 days
Onset	Sudden	Gradual
Fever	Present	Mild or absent
Other symptoms	General ill feeling, loss of appetite, nausea, abdominal discomfort, jaundice after several days	Wide range in severity—often includes loss of appetite, vague abdominal discomfort, nausea and vomiting, jaundice in several days
Prevention	General sanitation, proper sewage disposal, sterilization of needles, syringes, and other equipment, screening of blood donors, testing blood for transfusion, not getting tattoos, administration of gamma globulin to exposed persons	Same, except gamma globulin is not effective

Infectious Mononucleosis

Infectious mononucleosis is a viral infection centered in the lymph nodes. This disease is rarely fatal, but it often results in a period of general weakness that may last from one to several weeks. (There has been a tendency to overtreat this disease with prolonged restriction of activity, a practice which has actually slowed the recovery of many patients.) Other symptoms include fever, sore throat, and swollen lymph nodes. The production of atypical lymphocytes, a type of white blood cell, increases greatly. Many mild or symptomless cases occur in children. The disease is more severe among young adults.

The source of the virus is the nose and throat discharges of infected persons. It may be transmitted through direct contact or airborne droplets. Many persons continue to discharge the virus for as long as sixteen months following their recovery from the disease. No preventive methods are known.

Summary

I. Common Communicable Diseases

   A. Chickenpox

      1. Caused by the *varicella* virus

      2. No effective prevention yet available

   B. Common cold

      1. Caused by a variety of viruses

      2. No effective prevention yet developed

   C. Influenza

      1. Caused by a group of related viruses

      2. Vaccine available of moderate effectiveness

II. Diseases Entirely Preventable by Immunization

   A. Poliomyelitis

      1. Caused by three polio viruses

      2. Main vaccine in use is Sabin oral polio vaccine

   B. Smallpox

      1. Caused by highly contagious smallpox virus

      2. Vaccine contains the live virus of cowpox

   C. Measles

      1. Caused by the rubeola virus

      2. Vaccine contains the live, attenuated virus

D. Diptheria

    1. Caused by the bacillus *Corynebacterium diphtheriae*

    2. Immunizing agent is a toxoid: part of DPT series

E. Whooping cough

    1. Caused by bacterium *Bordetella pertussis*

    2. Immunization as part of DPT series

F. Tetanus

    1. Caused by bacterium *Clostridium tetani*

    2. Immunization as part of DPT series

G. German measles

    1. Caused by the rubella virus

    2. Vaccine contains live, attenuated rubella virus

H. Mumps

    1. Caused by the mumps virus

    2. Vaccine contains live, attenuated mumps virus

III. Some Other Important Diseases

  A. Tuberculosis

    1. Caused by bacillus *Mycobacterium tuberculosis*

    2. Best prevention is to maintain good general health and nutrition and avoid contact with known or suspected active cases

  B. Viral hepatitis

    1. Viral liver infections are a major problem today

    2. Two major diseases (compared in Table 2.3):

      a. Infectious hepatitis

      b. Serum hepatitis

  C. Infectious mononucleosis

    1. Caused by a virus

    2. No preventive methods are known

Questions for Review

1. What are "childhood diseases"? Can an adult catch them? Can they confer immunity?

2. Discuss the permanent aftereffects, if any, of measles, German measles, and mumps.

3. What is the most widespread infectious disease in the United States today? What are the chances of bringing this disease under control soon?

4. Are there any differences between influenza and the common cold? If so, what are they?

5. Which diseases are entirely preventable by immunization? Why do these diseases still exist?

6. Why is the Sabin oral polio vaccine used more often than the Salk vaccine? How do they differ?

7. What is DPT? How is it used? Is it for adults, children, or both?

8. Is tuberculosis still a major cause of death in this country? In other countries? Why or why not?

9. Describe the two methods used to check for the presence of tuberculosis.

10. Compare infectious hepatitis with serum hepatitis in terms of symptoms, sources of infection, and methods of prevention.

Chapter 3
VENEREAL DISEASES

The word "venereal" refers to Venus, the Roman goddess of love. A *venereal disease* (VD) is a disease that is mainly transmitted through sexual contact. Of the five venereal diseases recognized in the United States, two—gonorrhea and syphilis—are very common. The remaining three venereal diseases, chancroid, granuloma inguinale, and lymphogranuloma venereum are less common. Any of these diseases, however, can be very serious.

Why VD?

Except for having similar methods of transmission, the five venereal diseases are all different. What they do have in common is an affinity for the mucous membrances, such as those lining the reproductive organs, as well as relatively weak resistance to adverse environmental conditions such as dryness and cold. Transmission of the venereal disease generally requires the direct contact of warm, moist body surfaces. Sexual contact is ideal for this purpose.

No animal is known to carry any of the veneral diseases; the pathogens apparently evolved from harmless inhabitants of the human body or perhaps even of soil or water. Nor is it logical to view VD as punishment for "sin." Too many innocent people, such as newborn babies and spouses of unfaithful mates, are infected to make this idea plausible. It is best to think of the venereal diseases as potentially dangerous infections that happen to be commonly transmitted through sexual contact and should receive prompt treatment before others are infected or permanent damage results.

History of VD

The early history of the veneral diseases is obscured by the confusion and lack of knowledge that surrounded diseases in general until fairly recently. However, diseases fitting the descriptions of the venereal diseases can be traced back as far as 3,000 years. Hippocrates wrote of gonorrhea in 460 B.C., and several chapters of the Bible describe diseases which accurately correspond to the various stages of syphilis. The first recorded epidemic of syphilis swept through Europe late in the fifteenth century, possibly having been brought back from the New World by Columbus's crews. There was widespread death and disfigurement throughout much of Europe.

At one time gonorrhea and syphilis were thought to be the same disease. This erroneous idea was corrected in 1879 by the German bacteriologist Neisser, who identified the bacterium causing gonorrhea.

Both gonorrhea and syphilis have had a variety of names. Gonorrhea has been called "clap," "dose," "strain," and "G.C." Syphilis has been called "scab," "pox," "French pox," "Gallic disease," "Spanish sickness," "German pox," "Persian fire," "lues," and "syph." Syphilis received its present name in 1530 in a poem by a physician named Fracastoro about an afflicted Greek shepherd boy named Syphilus, who had offended the sun god.

Today's Incidence of VD

The number of cases of gonorrhea and syphilis exceeds the number of cases each year of strep throat, scarlet fever, mumps, measles, hepatitis, and tuberculosis *combined*. There are now well over 600,000 new cases of gonorrhea officially reported each year, but it is estimated that only one case out of every four actual infections is reported. For this reason, the actual incidence is probably more than 2.5 million per year, or one case out of every 100 people in the population. An estimated one-half million people in the United States suffer from untreated syphilis, and over 90,000 new cases are added each year.

Other studies indicate that even these estimates may be too conservative. For example, during the 12-month period ending June 30, 1973, gonorrhea screening programs cultured specimens from almost 5,000,000 women in the United States, of which 4.9 percent were positive for gonorrhea.*Although the highest gonorrhea rates (18.9 percent) were found predictably in visitors to venereal disease clinics, only 12 percent of the tests were performed in such clinics.

---

*Center for Disease Control, weekly morbidity and mortality report, October 12, 1973.

The remaining 88 percent were in other settings where typical gonorrhea rates included 2.3 percent of women visiting private physicians for all causes, 4 percent of women hospitalized for all causes, and 7.6 percent of women enrolling in manpower training programs. Few of these women were aware of their infection, as gonorrhea is symptomless in 80 to 90 percent of infected females.

Who Gets VD?

VD is in no sense a class phenomenon, that is, restricted to any one level in society. It has permeated all social levels; infections cross all lines of age, income, and ethnic group.

Most gonorrhea infections occur in the young, between the ages of 15 and 24. According to Dr. Walter Smartt, former chief of the Los Angeles County Venereal Disease Control Division, "the probability that a person will acquire VD by the time he's 25 is about 50 percent." Victims are, understandably, fairly equally divided between male and female. Yet, most *patients* are male because men more often show symptoms that lead to seeking of medical treatment. For every two women who are treated for gonorrhea, there are seven men treated. The difference is accounted for by the large number of undiagnosed females whose disease does not produce apparent symptoms (*asymptomatic*). Tests for gonorrhea conducted on female patients seeking treatment for purposes of birth control at public and private clinics indicate that about one in ten girls between the ages of 15 and 25 has gonorrhea and does not know it.

At least one in five persons in the United States with gonorrhea is under 20, and it has been diagnosed in youngsters under 9 years of age. Homosexuals are more apt to acquire gonorrhea than are any other identifiable group. Since homosexuals may change partners with frequency (50 contacts per month in some cases), and since the disease develops so quickly (two to five days after exposure), this infection spreads rampantly within the homosexual community. An estimated 50 percent of new cases of syphilis occur among male homosexuals.

Why the Increase in VD?

Throughout most of history, no specific cure for the venereal diseases was available. The introduction of sulfa drugs and penicillin in the 1940s promised a cure for both gonorrhea and syphilis with no more than a single office visit. Thus treatment moved from chronic care institutions into the private physician's office. Following the introduction of antibiotics, physicians began to rely solely on such treatment to eradicate VD. Treatment is vital because it may cure the infected individual. But it does not lead to the eradication of the disease from the population. (In the words of Dr. Smartt, "Treatment alone cannot, will not, and has never *eliminated* a communicable disease.")

After 1947, VD dropped steadily for a decade through the use of penicillin and other antibiotics. Then a blanket of complacency settled down over government agencies, the medical profession, and the public. Funds for VD control diminished, and VD began its spectacular resurgence. Late in the 1940s, patients were not even being interviewed for information on sexual contacts from or to whom the infection may have passed. Medical schools underemphasized its importance, and the general public became largely apathetic. Research on VD halted, there were few attempts to produce an appropriate vaccine or to develop a better method of diagnosing gonorrhea. Physicians were content to "spot-treat" isolated cases showing up in their offices. This neglect, particularly by the medical profession in developing better control procedures, is essentially the cause for the current gonorrhea epidemic (Figure 3.1).

According to some authorities, an important factor in the current VD epidemic is the birth control pill. "The Pill" has largely eliminated fear of pregnancy, thus encouraging greater freedom in sexual activity. Further, it has reduced the use of condoms, the only birth control method of value in preventing the transmission of VD. More than this, the Pill increases the alkalinity and moisture of the female genital tract, thus encouraging the rapid growth of gonorrhea organisms. Other contraceptive aids for females, such as vaginal jelly and foam, are acidic and thus provide an environment antagonistic to the growth of infectious organisms. The estimated risk of contracting gonorrhea for a woman engaging in a single act of unprotected intercourse with an infected partner is 40 percent; for a woman taking the Pill, it is almost 100 percent.

The lifestyles of young people have incorporated greater freedom of sex and greater personal mobility, both of which are favorable to the spread of VD. There are three other important changes in sexual behavior that may bear on the increase in incidence. They include (1) sexual relationships beginning at earlier ages, (2) greater variety in sexual partners, and (3) possibly less concern over the welfare of sexual partners.

Eradication of gonorrhea does not seem likely for some time due to several factors:

1. The so-called sexual revolution has had a profound influence and shows no signs of abating.
2. There are apparent weaknesses in the medical lines of defense. Some physicians still think either that VD, in the presence

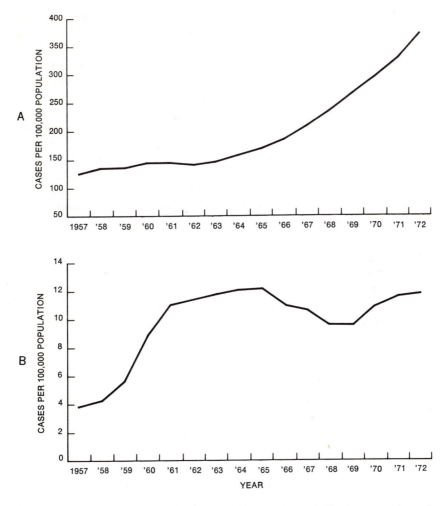

Figure 3.1 *Incidence of VD in United States, 1957–1972. A: gonorrhea; B: syphilis. Source: Center for Disease Control Morbidity and Mortality Report, 1972 Annual Supplement, July 1973.*

of penicillin, is no more significant than the common cold, or that VD patients are second-rate patients, and as such do not merit proper treatment. Many physicians are simply not aware of the possibilities in VD and the various forms it takes and do not *expect* their patients to get it.

3. The gonorrhea germ is constantly growing more resistant to penicillin. Treatment requires periodic increases in amount and use of different kinds of drugs for complete effectiveness.

4. The public attitude has been unconducive to control. It is extremely difficult to alter public attitudes, since there is a persistent association of VD and sex with "sin." Wittingly or unknowingly, there is constant reinforcement of the idea that VD is evidence of sexual transgression. Some people look upon the infected person as an undesirable member of society who is getting what he or she deserves.

5. There is no vaccine yet available for either syphilis or gonorrhea. The ideal preventive measure for VD would be a vaccine administered early in life. A vaccine for the prevention of syphilis is a possibility, but there has been little success to date in producing one. Because active immunity to gonorrhea is minimal (if it exists at all), a vaccine for the prevention of gonorrhea seems less likely than one for syphilis.

Gonorrhea

Gonorrhea is the *most common venereal disease* in the United States today. It is the second most common communicable disease in the United States, surpassed only by the common cold. Although less lethal than syphilis, gonorrhea is far more widespread and harder to control.

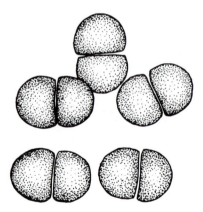

Figure 3.2   *Neisseria gonorrheae, the cause of gonorrhea.*

Gonorrhea is caused by a diplococcus called *Neisseria gonorrhoeae* (Figure 3.2), also called "the gonococcus." *Neisseria gonorrhoeae* is extremely selective about where it grows, requiring just the right temperature, humidity, and nutrients. It dies or is inactivated when exposed to cold or dryness. For this reason, the transmission of gonorrhea requires contact between warm, moist body surfaces. Inanimate objects such as toilet seats are of little importance in transmitting gonorrhea.

Source and Transmission

Humans are the only reservoir of gonorrhea. The organism occurs in the moist exudates from mucous membranes of infected persons. The gonococcus may be transmitted through various kinds of sexual contact—heterosexual or homosexual—including genital, oral-genital, and anal-genital.

Course of the Disease

Once the gonococcus gains a foothold, its symptoms in a male are entirely different from those in a female. In most males, infection is apparent in *two days to a week* after exposure; many, however, remain symptomless.

GONORRHEA IN THE MALE

The disease begins with a painful inflammation of the urethral canal in the center of the penis. This causes a scalding pain upon urination. The inflammation begins at the tip of the penis and works up the urethra. The result is a "drip" of pus from the penis. In early acute infection the discharge tends to be watery or milky. Later it becomes thick greenish-yellow, often tinged with blood.

The burning sensation upon urination may subside after two or three weeks. By this time the infection may have reached the prostate gland and testicles, as well as the bladder and kidneys. Permanent damage can include urinary obstruction, *chordee* (downward, painful curvature of the penis on erection), inflammation and abscesses of the prostate, or sterility due to blockage of the vas deferens and epididymis. Infection of the throat occasionally occurs following oral-genital contact. Such infections are especially common among homosexuals.

GONORRHEA IN THE FEMALE

Gonorrhea may produce no painful symptoms in women. In fact, about 80 percent of women infected do not realize they have the disease until their male partners discover their own infections. Infected women are therefore more likely to transmit the disease. The prevalence of asymptomatic carriers is an important part of the history of the gonorrhea epidemic. Public Health Service studies show that up to 5 percent of all women in the United States may be asymptomatic carriers of the gonococcus. Investigators are now reporting frequent discovery of gonococci in the urethras of males who reveal no symptoms.

The symptoms of gonorrhea in the female (when they exist) are different from those in the male. The usual symptom of a woman is irritation or "smarting" of the vagina accompanied by discharge. Unfortunately, such discharge is an unreliable sign in the female, since she may ordinarily experience vaginal discharges unrelated to gonorrhea. In the female the gonococcus prefers the cervix and fallopian tubes. In about 10 percent of cases the infection is found wholly in the rectum.

A gonorrhea infection generally moves methodically up the genital tract. In the vagina its effects are usually asymptomatic, or at least unclear. As it reaches the upper tract—the uterus, fallopian tubes, and ovaries—a pus discharge occurs and complications begin to set in, usually not until after at least one menstrual cycle. However, if the woman is on the Pill, complications may show up as quickly as 3–5 days after exposure.

GONORRHEA IN NEWBORN CHILDREN

Untreated gonorrhea in pregnant women may be responsible for *conjunctivitis* (an inflammation of the conjunctiva of the eye) in newborn children, acquired at the time of delivery. This condition is known as *ophthalmia neonatorum*. Infection of the infant's external genitalia may also result, especially in breech deliveries. In addition to the child, physicians have become infected when gonococcal-contaminated amniotic fluid has splashed into their eyes during a delivery.

COMPLICATIONS

Gonorrheal complications may include gonococcal arthritis, pelvic inflammatory disease (PID), abscesses in the fallopian tubes and ovaries, and a spilling over of pus material into the abdomen (giving rise to *peritonitis,* an inflammation of the inner lining of the abdominopelvic walls).

One study has shown that at least 12 percent of all females with gonorrhea suffer from some degree of invasion of the Fallopian tubes. This can result in sterility or ectopic pregnancy (a fertilized egg implanting itself in the fallopian tube rather than in the uterine wall) because of scar tissue which may block the free passage of the egg. Pus material may also collect into an abscess, which may rupture painfully. Gonorrhea-produced sterility is increasing and is presently the leading cause of sterility in the female.

Gonorrhea occasionally progresses into a serious, even fatal, systemic (blood-borne) infection. Systemic gonorrhea may attack the joints (causing arthritis), heart lining (causing endocarditis), heart muscle, brain, membranes covering the brain (causing meningitis), lungs, kidneys, veins, and skin. A common group of symptoms of systemic gonorrhea includes fever, arthritis, and sores on the skin. Even though the gonococcus is fragile outside the human body, its potential for tissue destruction and widespread complications within humans is great.

Diagnosis of Gonorrhea

A blood test has recently become available for the detection of gonorrhea. At the time of this writing its distribution is still limited and its effectiveness still being established. Other diagnostic methods involve demonstrating the presence of *Neisseria gonorrhoeae* organisms in stained microscope slides and in cultures on special growth media. For either slides or cultures, the sources of bacteria include swabs from the urethra of the male, cervix of the female, the anus, and the throat. Since females usually notice no symptoms of gonorrhea, periodic laboratory tests for gonorrhea are advisable even in the absence of symptoms if there is any chance of exposure to the disease.

Very often a patient may be infected with both syphilis and gonorrhea at the same time. While examining for gonorrhea, a physician should also be alert for symptoms of syphilis.

Treatment of Gonorrhea

The gonococcus has a long history of developing resistance to everything that has been used for its treatment. Some of the drugs that have gradually lost their effectiveness are potassium salts, silver compounds, sulfa drugs, and most recently, penicillin. Although penicillin is still the drug most commonly used against gonorrhea, much larger doses are now required than when the drug was first available. A typical dosage is now 4.8 million units of penicillin compared with 1.5 million units in the early 1960s. Even at this high level, penicillin often fails to cure gonorrhea completely. Fortunately, other drugs may be used when penicillin fails or the patient is hypersensitive (allergic) to penicillin.

It must be emphasized that *there is no effective home remedy for gonorrhea*. Nothing can be mixed up or bought from a drug store or by mail that will cure this or any other venereal disease. The infected person must see a private physician or his local public health department for effective treatment. It is most important that gonorrhea be treated promptly before any permanent damage, such as sterility, can occur.

Immunity to Gonorrhea

There is no vaccine that will prevent gonorrhea. Similarly, no immunity results from a case of gonorrhea. After a penicillin treatment wears off in a few days, reinfection can occur.

Syphilis

Syphilis is the *most serious* and the second most common venereal disease. Gonorrhea is normally a local surface infection, but syphilis is always a systemic infection. Their only similarity is that both are transmitted by sexual intercourse.

The organism causing syphilis is the spirochete (spiral bacterium) *Treponema pallidum* (Figure 3.3). This germ is very frail and cannot survive drying or chilling. It is killed within a few seconds after its exposure to air. Since the germ is so easily killed by air, it is easy to see why syphilis must be transmitted by sexual intercourse, kissing, or other intimate body contacts. The germ requires warm, moist skin or mucous membrane surfaces for its penetration into the body. After the spirochetes burrow through the skin or mucous membrane and enter the blood, they are carried throughout the body. Because its symptoms are so varied that they can resemble any one of many other diseases, syphilis has been called the "great imitator." It progresses through definite stages, which are explained in the following sections.

Figure 3.3   *Treponema pallidum, the cause of syphilis.*

Primary Syphilis

After infection with syphilis, there may be a symptomless incubation period of 10–90 days, although the usual period is 3–4 weeks. During this time the spirochetes multiply in the body.

The first symptom that appears is the *primary lesion* or *chancre* (pronounced "shanker"). This is a sore that appears at the exact spot where infection took place. The typical chancre (Figure 3.4) is pink to red in color, raised, firm, and painless. It is usually the size of a dime, but it may be so small that it resembles a pimple. The chancre is *swarming with spirochetes.* Any contact with it is likely to result in a syphilitic infection.

The usual location of the chancre is on or near the sex organs, but it can be on the lip, finger, or any part of the body. In females, the chancre is often within the vagina and, since it is painless, it goes unnoticed.

Even if primary syphilis is not treated (which it definitely should be), the chancre will disappear spontaneously in 3–6 weeks. But this disappearance of the chancre does not mean that the disease is cured. It is just progressing to the next stage. At about the time the chancre disappears, blood tests for syphilis become positive.

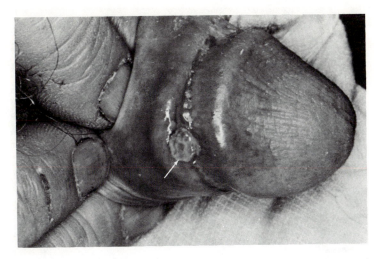

Figure 3.4 *Chancres are painless lesions, pink to red, raised, ulcerated, and firm. Chancre of the penis is shown here.*

Secondary Syphilis

In *secondary syphilis,* the true systemic nature of syphilis becomes obvious. Symptoms may appear throughout the body, starting 1–6 months after the appearance of the chancre, though in many cases this stage is skipped over. The most common symptom of secondary syphilis is a rash (Figure 3.5) that does not itch. This rash is variable in appearance and may cover the entire body or any part of it. Common sites of this rash are on the palms of the hands or the soles of the feet. Large, moist sores may develop on or around the sex organs or in the mouth. These moist sores are loaded with syphilitic germs. Contact with them, through sexual intercourse or even kissing, may cause syphilitic infection. Secondary syphilis is, therefore, extremely contagious.

Other symptoms that may occur in secondary syphilis include sore throat, headache, slight fever, red eyes, pain in the joints, and patches of hair falling out. When a person has these symptoms and thinks he may have been exposed to syphilis he should explain this fact to a physician. Because syphilis can easily be mistaken for one of many other diseases, it is difficult to diagnose. Without an accurate diagnosis, it may not be properly treated. Syphilis at this secondary stage is best diagnosed by means of specific blood tests for the disease.

The symptoms of secondary syphilis last from several days to several months. Then, like the chancre of primary syphilis, they disappear even without treatment. Syphilis has then entered the latent stage.

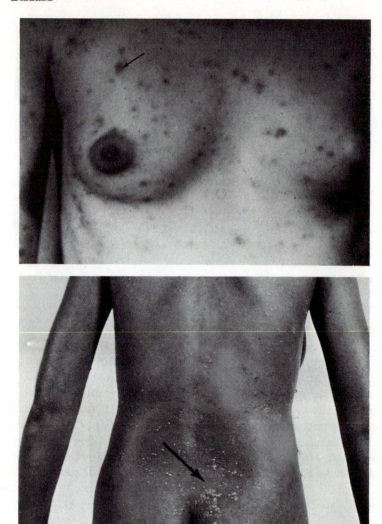

Figure 3.5 *Rash of secondary syphilis on breast and back.*

Latent Syphilis

Latency begins with the disappearance of untreated secondary symptoms; it may extend from a few months to a lifetime. Latency may be divided into two stages—a potentially infectious stage, *early latent syphilis,* and a noninfectious later stage, *late latent syphilis.*

EARLY LATENT SYPHILIS

If the disease remain untreated, there may be a series of recurring infectious lesions of the skin or mucous membranes for the first 2–4 years. Because of these new lesions the disease is considered communicable throughout its early latency. During the long latent period the disease loses some of its infectiousness; after the first two years, a person can rarely transmit syphilis through sexual intercourse, although a syphilitic pregnant woman can still transmit it to her unborn child (*congenital syphilis*) for an additional 2 years.

LATE LATENT SYPHILIS

When the individual has lost all ability to infect, the disease has entered the period of late latent syphilis, lasting anywhere from several months to a lifetime. During this period there are no discernible signs of illness. If routinely examined, the individual *will* show a positive blood test but will have no further signs. In this latent stage, progressive degeneration of the brain, spinal cord, hearing, sight, or bones may be occurring unnoticed. If and when the symptoms of this degeneration appear, the individual then slips into the last and most destructive stage.

Late Syphilis

Many people, having contracted syphilis *and* having allowed it, through neglect or ignorance, to progress untreated, may develop a late stage that will incapacitate or kill them. Although almost any part of the body may be affected, only the most common manifestations will be discussed below.

CARDIOVASCULAR SYPHILIS

The lesions in most cases of cardiovascular syphilis are located in the thoracic aorta. The elastic tissue is destroyed and the aorta stretches, producing an aneurysm. The infection may also involve the aortic valve, causing an insufficient flow of blood. The symptoms of cardiovascular syphilis do not differ from other heart and vascular disorders.

NEUROSYPHILIS

The symptoms of neurosyphilis arise from widespread destruction of brain tissue by large numbers of *Treponema pallidum*. The mental changes vary but most commonly become manifest in gradual changes of personality, decreased ability to work, and impairment of concentration and judgment. These changes produce abnormal behavior, including delusions, loss of memory, lack of insight, apathy or violent rages, convulsions, and disorientation. Neurosyphilis is responsible for many deaths, as well as for many of the chronic invalids seen in mental institutions.

IMPAIRED MUSCLE CONTROL

The most common outcome of the progressive destruction of the spinal cord by large numbers of spirochetes is impaired muscle control. Occasionally all reflexes may be lost, including the ability to vary pupil size (affecting vision), general sense of balance, and various elements of muscular coordination. Paresis (partial paralysis) may eventually result from untreated syphilis.

In treated cases life can be prolonged, but permanent care may be necessary because of extreme degeneration that may have taken place prior to treatment.

LOSS OF VISION

Syphilis can cause degeneration of the optic nerve, usually first noticed as a loss of peripheral vision. Central vision may be lost in advanced cases, leaving the individual completely blind.

Syphilis in Pregnancy

If a woman is infected with syphilis at the time of conception or shortly thereafter, the primary chancre appearing on her may be very mild or completely suppressed. Secondary symptoms in her skin are likely to be absent, and *if she has not had blood tests during her pregnancy* she may have no indication that she has syphilis until the birth of her child. Infection of a fetus takes place when the spirochetes of syphilis cross the placental membranes within the womb. Such infection of the fetus apparently does not occur before the fifth month of fetal life. Consequently, adequate treatment of a previously syphilitic pregnant woman *before the fifth fetal month* should insure the child's safety. Treatment given the mother after the fifth month may also cure the syphilitic fetus. Because of the conditions just discussed and because syphilis can also be acquired during pregnancy, blood tests during the first half of pregnancy and during the seventh month are considered adequate for detecting this disease.

In a majority of instances, infection of the fetus takes place quite late in pregnancy, and the more recent the mother's syphilitic infection, the greater probability that the child will be born with syphilis. A severe infection is very likely to lead to death of the fetus before birth, and syphilis is a common cause of stillbirth. Among the infants born alive to untreated syphilitic mothers, approximately 50 percent have syphilis at birth (congenital syphilis).

Congenital Syphilis

A syphilitic infant may show secondary lesions at birth, may appear normal at birth and develop lesions within a few months, or may remain without symptoms until adolescence, when the symptoms of late syphilis may appear. As a rule, the earlier the symptoms appear, the more severe the infection. Syphilis is capable of producing many different types of lesions, but never do all of them occur in one infant.

Of the various secondary lesions appearing at birth, *rhinitis*—an inflammation of the nose with a discharge of *Treponema pallidum* spirochetes—is most frequent. This discharge may interfere with breathing, is extremely infectious, and accounts for many infections of individuals who handle such children. If it is severe and continues over a long period, the growth of the nasal bones may be disturbed, resulting in the deformity known as "saddle nose" (Figure 3.6). Skin lesions at birth are frequent and are often similar to the rash seen in secondary stages of venereal syphilis. In a high proportion of children, the palms of hands, soles of feet, or skin about the mouth may be reddened, inflamed, and thickened at birth or shortly after birth. When this occurs around the mouth, fissures may radiate in all directions. After healing, these lesions and radiating scars about the mouth are known as *rhagades* (Figure 3.7).

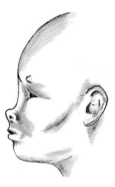

Figure 3.6   *Saddle nose, characteristic of congenital syphilis.*

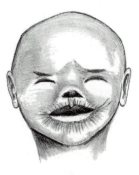

Figure 3.7   *Congenital syphilis, showing scars around the mouth (rhagades).*

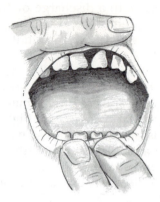

Figure 3.8   *Hutchinson's teeth, also characteristic of congenital syphilis.*

Following the secondary lesions, the course of untreated congenital syphilis is similar to that of venereal syphilis. These late symptoms may appear in a few months, at six or seven years of age, or in the late teens. Some of the more common are "Hutchinson's teeth" (Figure 3.8), which are "notched" or screwdriverlike permanent central incisors; *keratitis*, a condition of the eyes uncommon in young children but very common in older children and capable of causing permanent blindness; and injury to bones and body joints.

Diagnosis of Syphilis
Early diagnosis followed by prompt and adequate treatment can completely cure syphilis.

MICROSCOPIC EXAMINATION
The lesions of early syphilis are rich in *Treponema pallidum;* this fact provides the best means for conclusive diagnosis of the disease. *Treponema pallidum* taken from such a chancre of primary syphilis or from skin lesions of secondary syphilis can readily be seen under a microscope by what is termed "darkfield illumination."

BLOOD TESTS FOR SYPHILIS
Blood tests become positive only after a general invasion of the body by the spirochetes. The underlying principle of a blood test is appearance in the blood after syphilis infection (and occasionally following some other conditions) of an antibodylike substance called *reagin*. All of the blood tests for syphilis based on reagin in the blood are modifications of the original Wassermann test, an older test for determining blood reagin which was much less sensitive than present tests.

Besides the reagin tests, there are others for *Treponema pal-*

lidum spirochetes and specific antibodies produced by the body in response to syphilis infection. They are positive for syphilis only, are quite expensive, and involve complicated procedures that cannot be used as easily as the reagin tests for screening large numbers of individuals.

Syphilis Therapy

The purposes of treatment are to destroy all spirochetes, to initiate the healing of existing lesions, and to prevent further damage to the body. Treatment of syphilis also serves to prevent the spread of the disease to others. The earlier this treatment is begun, the more effective it is in accomplishing these purposes.

In the mid-1940s penicillin began to replace the lengthy, expensive, and difficult treatment of syphilis with arsenic products and bismuth preparations. Since that time the use of penicillin alone in the treatment of syphilis has become a worldwide standard.

The primary consideration in treatment is maintenance of a high penicillin level in the blood and tissues for a period of time sufficient to destroy all spirochetes present in the body. Consequently, treatment varies with progressive stages of the disease. Unfortunately, the widespread use of penicillin for treatment of a variety of other disorders has frequently added some difficulties to the diagnosis of syphilis. Syphilitic infection may be masked completely or its course altered by smaller doses of penicillin than are necessary to eliminate all the spirochetes. When a patient's allergy to penicillin precludes the use of this preferred drug, *erythromycin* and *tetracycline* are good alternatives. No matter what drug is used inadequate therapy may lead to a relapse. There is no home remedy, mail-order cure, or nonprescription drugstore product that will cure syphilis; it *must* have professional treatment by a physician.

Although no effective vaccine against syphilis has yet been developed, an immunity may sometimes develop in a person who has had the disease for several months or years before treatment. When syphilis is treated promptly (as it should always be), no immunity will develop, and reinfection can always take place if an individual is again exposed. The only reliable way to prevent syphilis is to avoid sexual contact with potentially infected persons. The *possibility* of infection is always present, no matter whom one has contact with; only the exercise of prudence in the choice of a sexual partner can diminish the *probability* of infection.

Other Venereal Diseases

Three other diseases are grouped with gonorrhea and syphilis as venereal diseases. These diseases occur throughout the world but are uncommon in most parts of the United States. Together, they amount to about 2,200 cases per year in the U.S., mainly in the Southern states.

Chancroid

Chancroid, also known as "soft chancre" or "soft sore," is an acute, localized, infectious disease usually acquired by sexual contact and caused by Ducrey's bacillus (*Hemophilus ducreyi*). About 3–5 days after exposure to the bacillus a small red area appears at the site of infection; this enlarges into a pimplelike growth that soon breaks down, forming an ulcer with ragged edges and exuding pus. If a cut or abrasion of the skin exists where contact with the bacillus is made, the lesion may appear within 24 hours. The ulcers bleed easily and are soft and very painful. A smear of the open ulcer is usually used by a physician to diagnose the disease.

In roughly half of all cases the disease is self-limiting and heals by itself. In the other half, in about a week the lymph glands near the ulcer may swell, accumulate large amounts of pus, and rupture spontaneously. Also, if a lesion is located in a body area that is hard to keep clean, is hidden, or does not receive proper treatment, rapidly destructive ulcerations (and occasionally giant ulcerations) can destroy much of the local tissue. The bacillus can be spread to adjacent areas of the body, causing reinfection and multiple lesions to develop. Systemic reactions are rare or mild, pain is the most frequent complaint, and extreme tissue destruction is the most severe complication. Chancroid ulcerations, for example, have been known to destroy the penis partially or completely.

Chancroid has been confused with the chancre stage of syphilis. Chancroid can be readily distinguished because its lesions are usually multiple and tender (instead of firm or hard) with a slightly grayish base. It is frequent companion to other venereal diseases such as gonorrhea, syphilis, and lymphogranuloma venereum. Tetracycline is used to treat chancroid, although alternative drugs such as sulfonamides, chloramphenicol, and streptomycin may also be used. The local cleansing of chancroid lesions with zephiran or antibiotic powders may also be useful. Chancroid is a disease of people who do not use soap and water frequently enough to keep the genital areas clean. The key to prevention of chancroid is cleanliness. The use of soap and water immediately after sexual exposure is a preventive measure.

There is some evidence that there are symptomless carriers of Ducrey's bacillus. Some women remain carriers of the disease and can transmit it to sexual partners after their own chancroidal lesions have healed, whereupon it is almost impossible to anticipate the danger of infection from them.

Granuloma Inguinale

Granuloma inguinale, the least common venereal disease, causes small, rounded, fleshy masses of pus-filled ulcerations that occur on skin covering the external genitals and inguinal (groin) region of the body. It occasionally spreads to the lymph nodes in the area. It is a chronic and progressive venereal disease, caused by a bacterium known as the Donovan body or *Donovania granulomatis*.

Little is known about the incubation period, which has been stated to be 8–12 weeks but has been known to run more than 100 days. The granulated ulcerations, most typical of the disease, usually are apparent by the fiftieth day after infection. The initial lesions appear on the genitals and slowly spread to the inguinal regions. The sore shows very little tendency to heal and spreads slowly but continuously. "Daughter" lesions frequently develop near the larger lesions. After several months, sometimes a year or more, the sores develop a sour-smelling, characteristic odor. The initial lesion takes the form of a deep red ulceration, and if the secondary lesions develop or if there is involvement of the lymph nodes, pain and fever may appear. Ultimately, in most untreated cases, the general health of the individual is impaired, anemia develops, and severe debility ends in death. When the disease is discovered and a diagnosis made, however, adequate treatment may bring about a complete cure. Tetracycline, given in doses of at least 2 grams daily for 15 days, is an effective remedy. Other drugs often used include chloramphenicol and streptomycin. Occasionally, dosages must be continued over a longer period of time to produce a cure.

Lymphogranuloma Venereum

Lymphogranuloma venereum is a sexually acquired infection of the lymph channels and lymph glands near the genital organs. It is a relatively common disease occurring throughout the world, especially in tropical and subtropical areas. It is found in the southern part of the United States, especially among lower socioeconomic groups.

The cause of lymphogranulom venereum is an extremely small bacterium, *Miyagawanella lymphogranulomatosis*. This organism is so small that it was for many years grouped with the viruses.

The primary lesion, an open ulceration, appears on the genital organs 5–21 days (7–12 days is most usual) after infection has taken place; it then vanishes very quickly. This lesion is often of such short duration that it escapes notice; thus the first symptoms of the disease may be swollen, hot, tender groups of lymph glands in the groin region, appearing 10–30 days after exposure. Fever, chills, headache, and joint pains may also be present. The inflamed lymph nodes frequently fill with pus and drain continuously. In females, the initial lesion is often internal or absent, and the first symptoms are enlarged lymph glands that appear near the rectum, where there are lymph glands that serve the vaginal area in which the disease is most likely to have started.

The course of the disease varies from one person to another. Some individuals may never be aware of the infection while in others the disease may progress for years, producing chronic lesions that may be so severe that the victim becomes an invalid. The diagnosis of lymphogranuloma venereum is by inoculating the pus from the lesions into laboratory animals to see if the infection is produced or by the Frei test, a skin test similar to the tuberculin test for TB. In the Frei test, an antigen is injected into the skin and if the person has the disease an inflammation appears around the site of the injection.

Antibiotics and sulfonamides are often used in treatment. Some evidence indicates that sulfonamides may be more effective. However, at the present time tetracycline in doses of 2 grams daily for 10 days or longer has proven to be effective in curing the disease. In some cases, extended dosages of any drug may be required.

Preventing the Venereal Diseases

So far, our discussion of venereal diseases has centered upon recognition of their symptoms and the importance of obtaining prompt treatment if infection occurs. But from both personal and public health standpoints, it is much more desirable to prevent any disease than to treat it. The prevention of the venereal diseases requires action by both the individual and public health personnel.

Personal Prevention

As with most other diseases, the ultimate responsibility for the prevention of the venereal diseases lies with the individual. The most important personal preventative measure is the avoidance of sexual contact with anyone who is *likely* to be infected with a venereal disease. Considering today's high incidence of venereal diseases, that would include anyone who has sexual contact with a variety of partners or who has sexual contact with another single sexual partner who, in turn, has a variety of sexual partners. Remember that venereal diseases can be transmitted through either heterosexual or homosexual contact and through either genital-genital, oral-genital, or anal-genital sex, and even through certain "petting" practices.

The prime mechanism for prevention of the venereal diseases, then, is selective sexual behavior. Unfortunately for the public as a whole, this mechanism has failed because it has never been widely practiced; the current VD epidemic is glaring evidence of this failure. Thus, for the person who chooses to be somewhat less discriminate

in his choice of sexual partners, it becomes important to make maximum use of other personal preventive (prophylactic) methods to
reduce the chances of infection. Note that we use the word "reduce"
rather than "eliminate," since even the best of the currently available
prophylactic methods are far from totally effective.

The single most important personal preventive method is probably the liberal use of soap and water immediately after sexual contact.
The pathogens of the venereal diseases that enter the body through
the skin can often be killed or removed in this manner. The three less
common venereal diseases, chancroid, lymphogranuloma venereum, and granuloma inguinale, can be almost entirely eliminated
by this simple technique.

Urination by a male immediately after sexual contact and prompt
douching by a female may help reduce the chance of infection with
gonorrhea. (It should be pointed out that douching is not effective as
a birth control measure and that frequent douching often results in
vaginal irritations and infections. Thus, douching should be reserved
for venereal disease prevention or for special situations upon the
recommendation of a physician.)

The use of a condom (rubber) over the penis of the male will help
prevent the transmission of VD, especially gonorrhea, in either
direction—from male to female or from female to male. To be effective, the rubber must be applied onto the erect penis at the very start
of any sexual activity, before any sexual contact is made. Even though
a condom is used, it is still important to wash with soap and water
immediately after contact because the condom covers only the penis,
and several of the venereal diseases, especially syphilis, can enter the
body through the skin at any point whatsoever. The condom thus
affords limited protection against syphilis. In its favor, however, it
should be noted that the condom is the only commonly used device
that is effective both as a prophylactic against gonorrhea and as a
contraceptive. Carefully and consistently used, it can be reasonably
effective for both purposes. Although it has traditionally been a male
responsibility to make sure of its availability for coitus, an enlight-
ened female might want to keep a supply of condoms available to
protect herself against VD and, if she is not otherwise protected,
against pregnancy as well.

Antibiotics have been used on a prophylactic basis, administered
either before or after possible exposure to VD, but this practice
cannot be recommended for routine use because it tends to breed
antibiotic-resistant strains of pathogens, including but not limited to
those which cause the venereal diseases, and because it tends to
build allergies to the antibiotics in those who receive them.

The ideal personal preventive would, of course, be a vaccine for each disease. Few communicable diseases have ever really been controlled until effective vaccines have been developed against them. Some progress has been made toward an effective vaccine against syphilis, but it has not yet reached a useful state. The prospects of an effective vaccine against gonorrhea seem especially dim, since no natural immunity to this disease develops, even after repeated infections.

Public Health Measures

Many methods are used by public health agencies in their fight against the venereal diseases, and, while VD is still rampant, it seems certain that incidence would be even greater than it is without the efforts of dedicated public health workers.

Most public health departments carry out programs of education concerned with prevention and symptoms of venereal diseases and the importance of prompt treatment. The media used often include newspapers, billboards, radio, TV, and posters in public places. Some public health departments assist local schools in their VD education programs, providing classroom materials and teacher training for effective VD instruction.

Clinics for the diagnosis and treatment of VD are also common functions of public health departments. The services of clinics are usually offered at little or no cost to the individual. Laws in most states have been revised to allow the treatment of minors, often as young as 12 years of age, without obtaining permission from their parents or otherwise notifying them. It has been found that when parental permission must be obtained prior to treatment, many young people will avoid treatment out of fear of reprisal from parents, thus tragically risking permanent damage from infection.

Another important public health function in VD control is case finding. In many localities, each patient treated for a venereal disease, especially for syphilis, is interviewed to determine from whom he might have caught the disease and to whom he might have transmitted it. These people can then be contacted, notified that they may be infected, and asked to visit the public health department or their private physician for VD testing. Since so many cases of VD are symptomless, this is the only way in which many infected people can learn of their disease before serious damage is done. Sometimes a patient is asked to name not only his sexual partners but any of his friends whom he feels might be infected.

One of the real barriers to effective case finding is that while by law every case of VD a physician treats must be reported to the local health department, in reality the majority of cases are not reported. The reporting rate for privately treated gonorrhea is especially low, even though gonorrhea reports are essentially for statistical purposes rather than for case finding. Many public health departments lack adequate funds for thorough case finding even for deadly syphilis.

While it may seem obvious, the VD patient should be warned to refrain from sexual contact with his previous partners until they have been tested and, if necessary, treated for VD. It is common (and frustrating) in VD clinics to find that a newly cured patient has gone back to the same partner who previously infected him and becomes reinfected again and again.

A technique that has revealed thousands of cases of syphilis is compulsory blood testing for certain people, such as applicants for marriage licenses, pregnant women, military personnel, hospital patients, and new employees of many corporations. Most of the cases so detected are in the symptomless latent period and, without detection and treatment, many would progress into late syphilis, with its irreversible damage to vital organs and even death.

It is an excellent idea for anyone who has a variety of sexual partners to obtain *an annual blood test for syphilis.* Many cases progress directly into the latent and eventually the late stages without ever exhibiting any noticeable symptoms. Yearly blood tests can reliably detect such cases, and the cost of such tests is minimal or even free if they are obtained through public health departments or free clinics.

In summary, while public health departments are making great efforts to control VD, syphilis and gonorrhea remain as epidemic diseases. It is imperative for the individual to take reasonable precautions against infection, to know the symptoms of these diseases, and to seek prompt treatment if these symptoms develop.

Summary

Venereal disease (VD)—transmitted mainly through sexual contact

I. Why VD?

    A. The five venereal diseases are all different

    B. Pathogens generally require close contact for transmission

    C. Not carried by animals

    D. Not punishment for "sin"

II. History of VD

    A. Early history uncertain

    B. Known for thousands of years

    C. Syphilis may have been carried from New World to Europe by Columbus's crews

III. Today's Incidence of VD

   A. Syphilis and gonorrhea are both very common today. Together exceed all other communicable diseases except common cold in incidence

   B. Exact incidence unknown—many cases unreported

   C. Current estimates:

      1. 2.5 million cases of gonorrhea per year in U.S.

      2. 90,000 new cases of syphilis per year

      3. 500,000 people in U.S. with untreated syphilis

   D. Recent (1973) screening of 5,000,000 women showed 4.9 percent positive for gonorrhea

IV. Who Gets VD?

   A. Could be anybody

   B. High rates in young people

   C. High rates in homosexuals

V. Why the Increase in VD?

   A. Birth control pill reduced use of condoms, also changed environment of vagina to favor gonorrhea

   B. Changing lifestyles:

      1. Sexual relationships at earlier ages

      2. Greater variety in sexual partners

      3. Less concern over welfare of sexual partners

   C. Physicians often not VD-conscious

   D. Growing resistance of gonorrhea to penicillin

   E. Public attitude toward VD as deserved punishment for "sin"

   F. Lack of effective vaccines

VI. Gonorrhea

   A. Most common VD in the U.S

   B. Caused by diplococcus *Neisseria gonorrhoeae,* a very delicate organism

   C. Source and transmission:

      1. Humans only reservoir

      2. Transmitted through any kind of sexual contact

   D. Course of the disease

      1. Gonorrhea in the male

         a. Most develop symptoms, though many remain symptomless.

         b. Begins as infection of urethra

     c. May progress to prostate, vas deferens, epididymis, and testes

     d. Blockage of vas deferens may cause sterility

     e. Throat infections common among homosexuals

  2. Gonorrhea in the female

     a. Usually no symptoms

     b. Moves up through reproductive organs

     c. May lead to sterility through scarring of fallopian tubes

  3. Gonorrhea in newborn children—may cause eye infection

  4. Complications

     a. Arthritis

     b. Pelvic inflammatory disease (PID)

     c. Attack of various internal organs

E. Diagnosis

  1. Newly available blood test

  2. Microscope slides

  3. Cultures

F. Treatment

  1. Organism develops resistance to each drug used

  2. Treated with penicillin and other antibiotics

  3. No effective home remedy is available

G. Immunity

  1. No vaccine yet available

  2. Repeated infections may occur—no immunity develops

VII. Syphilis

A. The most serious venereal disease

B. Caused by spirochete called *Treponema pallidum*

C. Always a systemic disease

D. Progresses through definite stages:

  1. Incubation period of 10–90 days

  2. Primary syphilis—chancre at site of infection

     a. May be anywhere on body

     b. Swarming with spirochetes

  3. Secondary syphilis—symptoms throughout body

     a. Rash (variable in appearance)

     b. Sores in mouth and on sex organs (loaded with spirochetes)

       c. Sore throat, headache, slight fever, pain in joints, patches of hair falling out

       d. May last from several days to several months

    4. Latent syphilis—no symptoms

       a. May last from a few months to a lifetime

       b. Early latent syphilis

          (1) First 2–4 years

          (2) Secondary symptoms may recur from time to time

       c. Late latent syphilis

          (1) No outward symptoms

          (2) Only transmission possible is from mother to fetus

    5. Late syphilis—permanent damage to vital organs

       a. Heart and blood vessels

       b. Nervous system:

          (1) Behavior changes

          (2) Impaired muscle control, paralysis

          (3) Loss of vision

E. Syphilis in pregnancy—fetus may be killed or severely damaged (congenital syphilis)

F. Diagnosis of syphilis:

    1. Microscopic examination for presence of spirochetes

    2. Blood tests

G. Treatment—usually penicillin

VIII. Other Venereal Diseases

  A. Chancroid

    1. Caused by bacillus *Hemophilus ducreyi*

    2. Produces painful, destructive lesions of sex organs

    3. Easily preventable with soap and water

  B. Granuloma inguinale

    1. Caused by *Donovania granulomatis* (small bacteria)

    2. Chronic, progressive disease

  C. Lymphogranuloma venereum

    1. Caused by extremely small bacteria

    2. Severity ranges from mild to very serious

IX. Preventing Venereal Disease

  A. Personal prevention

    1. Avoid sexual contact with persons likely to be infected

    2. Soap and water after sexual contact

    3. Condom (rubber)

  B. Public health measures

    1. Education

    2. Public VD clinics

    3. Case finding

Questions for Review

1. What do syphilis and gonorrhea have in common? In what ways do they differ?

2. What is believed to be the origin of the venereal diseases?

3. What is the approximate incidence of gonorrhea and syphilis?

4. What are some possible causes of the current VD epidemic?

5. In what ways have birth control pills contributed to the incidence of gonorrhea?

6. What shape of bacteria are responsible for gonorrhea? For syphilis?

7. In addition to the sex organs, where else may gonorrhea infections occur?

8. How are syphilis and gonorrhea diagnosed?

9. What are the most likely symptoms of gonorrhea in the male? In the female?

10. What is meant by the statement that syphilis is always a systemic disease?

11. Outline the stages of syphilis, giving the symptoms and approximate duration of each stage.

12. Discuss methods of personal prevention of VD. Public health preventive measures.

Chapter 4
NON-COMMUNICABLE DISEASES

In the previous chapters we dealt with the communicable diseases—those diseases caused by infectious agents that can be passed directly or indirectly from one person to another. In this and the following chapters, we will consider some of the more important *noncommunicable diseases*—those that are not communicated from one person to another.

Importance of Noncommunicable Diseases

Throughout most of the course of history, the principal causes of death were the communicable diseases. In some parts of the world, this is still the case. But during the first half of the twentieth century, advances in preventive medicine have vastly altered the pattern of disease in the United States and many other countries. In 1900 the leading causes of death in this country were tuberculosis and pneumonia—both communicable diseases. Today these diseases are of secondary importance, and their places are now occupied by the *cardiovascular diseases*, the number one cause of death, and *cancer*, the number two cause.

Table 4.1 indicates this change. Improvements in diagnosis, treatment, sanitation, nutrition, housing, and working conditions, as well as more specific preventive measures, such as immunizations, have played important roles in the conquest of the communicable

TABLE 4.1   Leading Causes of Death in the United States—1900 and 1975

1900 (Life expectancy 46.3 years for males, 48.3 years for females)		1975 (Life expectancy 67.1 years for males, 74.8 years for females)	

RANK	CAUSE	RANK	CAUSE	PERCENT OF ALL DEATHS
1	Tuberculosis	1	Heart and circulatory disorders	51%
2	Pneumonia	2	Cancers, all types	18%
3	Intestinal infections	3	Accidents	6%
4	Heart diseases	4	Pneumonia and influenza	3%
5	Diseases of infancy	5	Diabetes	2%

diseases. Drugs, such as antibiotics and sulfas, have greatly reduced communicable diseases, even as other public hazards, such as those in lower economic areas of our large cities, have remained.

The increase in noncommunicable disease has been due in large part to the increased average life span. In just 100 years, from 1860 to 1960 the proportion of persons in the United States over 45 years of age climbed from 13 percent to 29 percent of the population. This increase in older age-groups is currently changing the whole field of preventive medicine. Whereas previous efforts were directed largely toward the control of communicable diseases of early life, efforts are now being directed increasingly toward the noncommunicable diseases common in middle and later life.

Arthritis

Arthritis is a general term for any inflammation of the joints. Its symptoms commonly include stiffness in the joints and mild to extreme pain, especially when affected joints are moved. With some types of arthritis, the joints become twisted and deformed.

About 100 types of arthritis are known today. Among the more important forms are *osteoarthritis* (degeneration of the joint) and *rheumatoid arthritis* (inflammation and swelling of the joint). A less common form, *gout,* is the painful deposit of urate crystals in and around the joints.

Arthritis is the number one crippler in the United States today. Over 17 million people suffer from some form of arthritis. For more than 3 million of these people, the symptoms are severe enough to limit their activity. Arthritis becomes more common and more severe as people grow older. Over 80 percent of people over age 65 are affected by some degree of arthritis. Rheumatoid arthritis is also fairly common among younger people. The measurable cost of arthritis in this country, including treatment and loss of earning power, is over 4 billion dollars a year.

Considerable progress has been made in the treatment of arthritis. While there is still no permanent cure for most forms of arthritis, many victims who five years ago would have been immobilized or restricted drastically in their activity can now enjoy a normal life. Treatment involves drugs, directed at both the basic cause of the problem and the relief of pain; total joint replacement with joints of plastic and metal; and a variety of less drastic surgical methods. Bed rest, special exercises, and possibly acupuncture, all under medical supervision, may help in mild forms of arthritis. Early detection and treatment of arthritis is important in the prevention of its progression into a crippling form.

It is important to consult with a reputable physician for the treatment of arthritis. One of the most prevalent forms of quackery today is the dispensing of fraudulent or unproven treatments for arthritis. This field is lucrative to quacks because of the great numbers of people affected and the fact that no complete cure yet exists for many types of arthritis. Arthritic persons should be cautioned to avoid unproven treatments, whether sold by mail order, in stores, or administered by unethical practitioners.

Diabetes

Diabetes mellitus is a disturbance of the metabolism (body chemistry), resulting from a deficiency of the hormone *insulin*. Insulin is produced in the pancreas by special clusters of cells called the *islets of Langerhans*. Insulin has the important function of increasing the rate of movement of glucose (blood sugar) through the membranes of most of the cells of the body. In diabetes, the blood sugar is unable to enter the cells in adequate amounts.

The tendency toward diabetes may be transmitted through recessive genes. Not everyone who inherits the genes for diabetes actually develops the disease, however. Diabetes is most common among older people, especially those who are overweight. Less commonly, it is a problem during youth. Diabetes developing during childhood, called *juvenile-onset* diabetes, is usually much more severe than diabetes developing in adults. Many adults who carry the hereditary makeup for diabetes can avoid the disease entirely by merely controlling their food consumption.

Between 1 and 2 percent of the population of the United States is definitely known to suffer from diabetes, but surveys in which large numbers of persons have been tested for diabetes have shown that its true incidence may be closer to 4 percent of the population. This indicates that many people have this dangerous disease without even knowing it. Periodic testing for diabetes is important for everyone, especially for relatives of known diabetics.

There may or may not be noticeable symptoms of diabetes. The most common symptoms that do appear include frequent urination, excessive thirst, craving for sweets and starches, and weakness. The most common medical test for diabetes is analysis of the urine for the presence of sugar. If sugar is present, a test is made for the level of sugar in the blood. The blood-sugar level is abnormally high in diabetics, a condition called *hyperglycemia.*

Some cases of adult-onset diabetes can be controlled with modification of the diet or increased exercise. The diet should be lower than average in carbohydrates (sugars and starches). Exercise increases the movement of blood sugar into muscle cells, thus helping to control the disease.

Many cases of diabetes, particularly those of juvenile-onset, require treatment with insulin or other drugs. For many years insulin was the only effective drug for the treatment of this disease. If the dosage of insulin is properly balanced with the intake of carbohydrates, most of the consequences of diabetes can be prevented. This is not a cure for the disease, merely a control. The drug must be taken indefinitely.

One disadvantage of insulin is that it must be taken by injection since, being a protein, it is digested if taken by mouth. Several other drugs are available which can be taken by mouth. These drugs stimulate the cells of the pancreas to produce insulin. Such drugs are effective only in adult-onset diabetics whose cells have retained some ability to produce insulin. If this ability has been totally lost, as in many severe juvenile-onset cases, insulin by injection is still the only effective treatment.

If diabetes is not adequately controlled, severe dehydration and acidity of the body fluids may occur. The result may be *diabetic coma* (unconsciousness) which is almost always fatal unless the patient receives immediate medical treatment. The breath smells of acetone and breathing is rapid. Another situation that requires immediate medical treatment is *insulin shock,* the result of an overdose of insulin. In insulin shock, the blood-sugar level is too low (*hypoglycemia*) for proper functioning of the central nervous system. As the blood-sugar level drops progressively lower, the person first trembles and seems nervous, then goes into convulsions, and finally drops into a state of coma. This coma can be distinguished from the diabetic coma by the absence of acetone breath and rapid breathing.

If an overdose of insulin has been administered to a diabetic and he is still conscious, sugar or some product containing sugar, such as candy or orange juice, should be given to him. If he is already unconscious, he should receive immediate medical attention.

In addition to diabetic coma, untreated diabetes may lead to early death from heart disease or infection, or to blindness, kidney disease, stillbirth, or infant death of babies born to diabetic women.

They key steps in preventing such damaging results of diabetes are, in summary:

1. *Avoid becoming overweight.* This alone will prevent many potential cases of diabetes from ever developing.

2. *Have periodic medical examinations* that include blood or urine tests for diabetes.

3. *Seek medically supervised treatment* of a diagnosed case, including proper diet, exercise, and drugs.

A much less common condition, *diabetes insipidus,* results from improper functioning of the posterior lobe of the pituitary gland. Damage to the posterior pituitary is usually the result of an injury or a disease, such as syphilis. The antidiuretic hormone (ADH) release by this gland is suppressed, causing excessive production of urine (polyuria). Unless water is continually replaced, dehydration develops rapidly, leading to acidosis, unconsciousness, and death.

Noncommunicable Respiratory Disorders

Severe respiratory disorders are among the most disabling of human diseases since they interfere with the oxygen supply that is so vital to all living tissues. The noncommunicable respiratory disorders, such as asthma, chronic bronchitis, and emphysema, therefore rank high as causes of human discomfort, disability, and death.

Asthma

Asthma is a disease in which there are periodic attacks of difficulty in breathing. During an attack, wheezing and shortness of breath may be mild or so severe as to require medical treatment in order to prevent death.

The choked breathing that accompanies an asthma attack is caused by a narrowing of the *bronchioles,* small tubes inside the lungs (Figure 4.1). This narrowing can be the result of a swelling of the membrane that lines the bronchioles, a spasm (constriction) of the tubes, or mucus blockage of the tubes.

There are many causes of asthma, among which allergic reactions are prominent. Asthma related to allergy is called *extrinsic asthma.* About 75 percent of the people who have asthma are allergic to one or more substances. Many cases of asthma are associated with

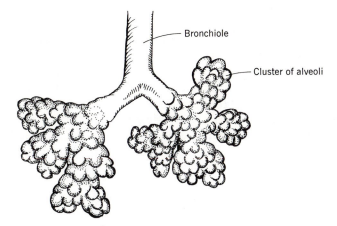

Figure 4.1 *Microscopic structure of the lungs. Each lung consists of millions of microscopic air sacs (alveoli) supplied with air by small ducts (bronchioles).*

bacterial infections of the sinuses, throat, and nose (*instrinsic asthma*). Most of these cases improve if the infection clears up. In some asthmatic patients, attacks are brought on or made worse by emotional stress that may lead to constriction of the bronchioles.

It is important that asthma sufferers receive the best available medical treatment, since prolonged or repeated attacks can cause permanent damage to the lungs and heart. Forced breathing can stretch the lung tissue, leading to the very serious condition known as *emphysema,* to be discussed below.

The treatment of asthma must be under the supervision of a physician. No one should try to diagnose or treat himself. The exact cause of the attacks must be determined in order to decide the proper type of treatment. If an allergy is involved, the substance causing the allergy can sometimes be avoided, or, in some cases, the patient can be desensitized by a series of injections. If an infection is involved, it should be promptly treated. Ways may have to be found to reduce emotional stress, if this is the cause of the attacks. A change of climate may or may not be useful. The decision to move to another area should be made only after consultation with a physician. Various drugs are prescribed to provide relief from asthma attacks.

Chronic Bronchitis

The inside of the bronchiole is lined with a highly specialized membrane (see Figure 1.10). This membrane secretes a layer of mucus to trap the foreign matter that enters the lungs. Millions of hairlike cilia constantly sweep the layer of mucus with its trapped foreign particles upward to the throat where it is swallowed.

Repeated irritation of this ciliated mucous membrane can paralyze the action of the cilia, eventually destroy them, and stimulate excessive production of mucus. This is the condition known as *chronic bronchitis.* Since the cilia can no longer clear the lungs of mucus, it accumulates until the flow of air through the bronchioles is obstructed. This obstruction then triggers a spell of coughing that helps clear the lungs. Frequent coughing is the most prominent symptom of chronic bronchitis. Other symptoms may include shortness of breath and wheezing.

Frequent coughing caused by chronic bronchitis may gradually stretch and tear the minute air sacs of the lungs (*alveoli*), creating emphysema.

The main treatment of chronic bronchitis consists of eliminating the irritation that causes it. The source of irritation is often a chronic infection or smoking tobacco. The so-called smoker's cough is in reality a symptom of chronic bronchitis. The first step in treating any lung disorder is to *stop smoking.* If the source of irritation is an infection, this should receive prompt treatment. Coughing itself can contribute to the irritation of the bronchioles, thus creating a self-perpetuating condition. Coughing should be avoided unless absolutely necessary, and then it should be as gentle as possible. Above all, chronic bronchitis should receive the treatment of a physician.

Emphysema

Emphysema is a deterioration of the lungs that develops gradually over a period of years. It is therefore more common among older persons, although it may begin to develop during youth. In emphysema, the thin walls of the tiny air sacs lose their elasticity and tear. This reduces the ability of the lungs to exhale.

The lungs swell up permanently, creating a "barrel chest" appearance in the victim of emphysema. Exhaling becomes extremely slow and difficult. The blood circulates with difficulty through the damaged lung tissue, creating a great burden on the heart, which must pump all the blood through the lungs before it can circulate to the body. Emphysema is an extremely disabling disease and often leads to fatal heart failure.

The development of emphysema often can be traced to prolonged asthma or chronic bronchitis. The most common link between emphysema victims is a history of heavy smoking. The disease is far more common among smokers than among nonsmokers. Air pollution and metabolic disorders are also believed to be associated with emphysema.

There is no real cure for emphysema. A physician may prescribe certain measures, such as mild exercise, drugs, and special breathing techniques, but these mainly help the patient to live with his condition; they do not cure it.

Occupational Diseases

Occupational diseases are diseases that result from occupational exposure to some harmful element. Such elements may be physical, chemical, or biological. Some occupational diseases are specific to given occupations and do not occur among the general public; others which do occur in the general population may be considered occupational diseases if their incidence is greatly increased within a given occupation.

Despite considerable improvement in working conditions during the past 50 years, occupational diseases still plague workers in many industries. In some cases the hazards, such as black lung in miners as a result of breathing coal dust, have been known for many years. Many corporations show little concern for the health of their employees or may lack the technical ability or economic strength to overcome occupational hazards. Other occupational hazards, such as asbestos dust and polyvinyl chloride, have become known more recently and intensive corrective programs are now underway. And there are undoubtedly other serious occupational health hazards that are still undiscovered.

Chemical Hazards

Many occupational diseases result from exposure to chemical substances, such as solvents, dusts, and gases. Almost every occupation involves some exposure to potentially dangerous chemicals. Even an office worker may be exposed to such solvents as type cleaners and duplicating fluids. Employers vary in the degree of protection they provide their employees against dust, vapor, and other forms of chemicals. Employees may also fail to follow the safety precautions outlined for them. People often believe, erroneously, that as long as no immediate effects are noticed, no harm is being done. Many chemicals, such as asbestos, may result in cancers which appear many years following exposure.

Physical Hazards

Certain physical factors, such as temperature, noise, and radiation, may produce occupational diseases. The effects of temperature extremes depend on how high or low the temperature is, the humidity, the length of exposure, and the degree of exertion taking place.

Exposure to loud noise, such as that which occurs in many places of employment, may cause temporary or permanent hearing loss. Permanent damage is cumulative and reaches its maximum after 5–10

TABLE 4.2   Intensity of Common Sounds

Sound	Intensity in Decibels
Human whisper	30
Normal conversation	60
City traffic	80
Garbage disposal unit	80
Domestic quarrel	80
Vacuum cleaner	85
Garbage truck	85
Food blender	93
Subway train	95
Jackhammer	95
Power lawnmower	96
Printing press	97
Farm tractor	98
Punch press	105
Boiler shop	105
Motorcycle	110
Riveting gun	110
Rock band (amplified)	114 to 140
Jet airplane	135 to 150
Siren	150

Source: *Medical World News*, Vol. 10, No. 24; pp. 42–47, June 13, 1969, and other sources.
Note: A decibel is the smallest difference in intensity of sound that the human ear can detect. The scale is logarithmic; a difference of 10 decibels represents a tenfold increase in sound intensity.

years of exposure. The degree of hearing loss depends upon the pitch (frequency) of the sound and its intensity measured in decibels. Damage begins to occur at 90–120 decibels, depending on the pitch. Some typical noise intensities are listed in Table 4.2.

Radiation presents a particular hazard in that it cannot be detected by any of the human senses—it is colorless, odorless, noiseless, and painless. Thus radiation levels must be monitored by instruments, and employees must be particularly careful to follow all safety precautions. Some of the harmful effects of radiation are listed in Table 4.3.

Biological Factors

Some jobs, especially in agriculture, expose a person to infectious disease agents (pathogens). Diseases such as brucellosis and anthrax can be contracted from animals or animal products. Certain lung-invading fungi, such as histoplasmosis and coccidioidomycosis, are commonly contracted by agricultural or construction workers through exposure to airborne spores of the fungi in dust.

TABLE 4.3   Effects of Exposure to Radiation

Form of Radiation	Effects
Ionizing radiations: Gamma rays X rays	Damage genetic material of cells, causing mutations, cancers, or death of cells. Any tissue of body may be damaged. Large doses always fatal.
Ultraviolet rays	Little penetrating ability. Affect only skin and eyes. Burn skin, produce tanning, thicken and age skin, cause skin cancer. Cause inflammation of conjunctiva of eye, clouding and ulcers of cornea (usually temporary), clouding of lens (cataract; not proven).
Intense visible light	Causes inflammation of conjunctiva and cornea, temporary or permanent loss of vision through damage to retina.
Infrared rays	Cause burning of skin, temporary or permanent damage to retina of eye, possible cataracts.
Laser beams	Cause skin burns, heat injury to any part of eye.
Microwaves (radar and others)	Main effect is production of heat in tissue where absorbed. Produce cataracts.

Eliminating Occupational Hazards

Many corporate executives and other employers have come to realize that the health of their employees has a great influence on profits. An experienced, vigorous employee is worth much more to an employer than either the same person weakened by an occupational disease or an inexperienced replacement, needed if the employee becomes completely disabled. But many employers must be motivated to show concern for their personnel. The employees themselves should be alert to hazards, pointing them out to management and refusing to risk further exposure if conditions are not corrected. Employee groups, such as unions, can often successfully bring pressure to correct hazardous working conditions. Finally, strict industrial safety laws are on the books and are now being vigorously enforced under the OSHA (Occupational Safety and Health Act) at the federal level and by many states.

Summary

I. Noncommunicable Diseases

  A. Diseases that are not transmitted from one person to another

  B. Advances in preventive medicine have altered the pattern of communicable and noncommunicable diseases

   1. Incidence of communicable disease has declined in the United States as the result of improvements in personal and community health, diagnosis, treatment, and immunization

   2. Incidence of noncommunicable diseases has increased in the United States because of the increased average life span

II. Arthritis

  A. Inflammation of the joints

  B. Many types

  C. Number one crippler in United States today

  D. Progress being made in treatment

  E. Early detection and treatment important

III. Diabetes

  A. Hereditary tendency probably transmitted through recessive genes

  B. Deficiency of insulin resulting in disturbance of body chemistry is diabetes mellitus

  C. Blood-sugar level is abnormally high in diabetics

  D. Symptoms may include frequent urination, excessive thirst, craving for sweets and starches, and weakness

  E. Urine test for presence of sugar

  F. Many cases require treatment with insulin; some can be controlled with modifications in diet or increased exercise

  G. Diabetic coma—uncontrolled diabetes results in unconsciousness which is almost always fatal

  H. Insulin shock—overdose of insulin

  I. Preventive measures:

   1. Avoid becoming overweight

   2. Have periodic medical examinations

   3. Seek medically supervised treatment

  J. Diabetes insipidus the result of inadequate production of antidiuretic hormone by posterior lobe of pituitary gland

IV. Noncommunicable Respiratory Disorders

  A. Asthma

   1. Attacks of difficulty in breathing

2. Allergy reactions are prominent

3. Proper treatment can reduce or eliminate serious effects in many cases

B. Chronic bronchitis

    1. Excessive production of mucus in bronchioles caused by irritation of ciliated mucous membrane

    2. Source of irritation is often smoking

C. Emphysema

    1. Gradual deterioration of lungs

    2. Tiny air sacs in lungs lose elasticity and tear

    3. Creates a great burden on the heart

    4. Asthma, chronic bronchitis, and smoking are common links to emphysema

    5. Mild exercise, drugs, and special breathing techniques prescribed by physician may help patient live with disease, but will not cure it

V. Occupational Diseases

A. Despite improvements of past 50 years, still a problem in many industries

B. Chemical hazards

    1. Some exposure in almost every occupation

    2. Effects may not become apparent for many years

C. Physical hazards

    1. Temperature extremes

    2. Loud noise—causes permanent loss of hearing

    3. Radiation—many serious effects

D. Biological factors (pathogens)—from exposure to animals or dust

E. Eliminating occupational hazards

    1. Some employers take the initiative

    2. Others need motivation by employees, unions, government agencies

Questions for Review

1. Distinguish between communicable and noncommunicable diseases.

2. Why have noncommunicable diseases replaced communicable diseases as the leading causes of death in the United States?

3. What is arthritis? What are some major types?

4. Diabetes is the result of a hormone deficiency in the body. What is the hormone? What is its function?

5. What are the three key steps in prevent the damaging results of diabetes?

6. What is the most common cause of asthma?

7. How does chronic bronchitis develop? How is it treated? What is the relationship between chronic bronchitis and the so-called smoker's cough?

8. What is the relationship between emphysema and chronic bronchitis? Has a common cause for emphysema been identified? Can emphysema be cured?

Chapter 5

CARDIOVASCULAR DISEASES

In the early 1900s the greatest concern of physicians in the United States was with certain infectious diseases—tuberculosis, pneumonia, diarrhea, typhoid fever—and with malnutrition. Gradually the picture has changed. Today the control of most infectious diseases has been virtually mastered with the help of antibiotics, vaccines, and effective control measures by public health departments.

But to date, modern medicine has been unable to conquer certain noncommunicable diseases. Circulatory and heart diseases, which were the number four cause of death in terms of incidence in 1900, are now the *number one* cause among all age groups. These diseases account for over 50 percent of all deaths in the United States today.

As noted in Chapter 4, one reason for the increase in incidence of circulatory diseases is that, with the conquest of certain communicable diseases, life expectancy has increased. This, in turn, has increased people's chances of developing circulatory diseases at a later age. Aspects of the American way of life not present in societies with lower incidence of heart disease appear to relate to this higher incidence—the stresses of personal accomplishment, diets high in saturated fats, the tendency toward obesity with age, lack of sufficient physical exercise, and the high incidence of smoking.

The aim of medicine today is not simply to understand the nature of these diseases and to treat those afflicted, but to prevent such diseases in those not yet afflicted.

This chapter will examine the structure and functions of the circulatory system, its most common disorders, and the current knowledge derived from heart research.

Circulation

The body consists of billions of cells. In order to function properly, the masses of cells must receive adequate food, water, and oxygen. As a result of their chemical activities, they produce waste products that must be removed from the body. Certain cells, such as those in the glands, produce essential secretions required by other parts of the body, and such secretions must be transported throughout the body.

Thus the body requires some form of overall transportation system that will reach all of the cells quickly and efficiently. The *circulatory system* (Figure 5.1) is responsible for such continuous and rapid movement of foods and wastes to and from the cells.

Blood

The purpose of blood is transport. In circulation, blood is directed to the lungs, where it obtains the oxygen it carries to the body cells. The blood picks up wastes from the cells and carries them to the kidneys, where they are excreted. Digested foods are picked up from the digestive tract and carried to the cells for immediate use or storage. Chemicals called *hormones* (secreted by specific glands) are carried throughout the body to regulate and coordinate body activities. Blood also regulates body temperature and carries substances that protect the body against disease.

Components of Blood

Under normal conditions blood consists of a straw-colored fluid, or *plasma,* in which are suspended corpuscles—red blood cells (*erythrocytes*) and white blood cells (*leukocytes*)—and platelets. (See Figure 5.2.) Plasma makes up about 55 percent of the whole blood, and the cellular parts make up about 45 percent. Since blood is continuously exchanging materials with the tissues (groups of cells), its composition is constantly changing.

PLASMA

This liquid portion of blood is about 90 percent water. The remaining 10 percent consists of many different substances, including proteins,

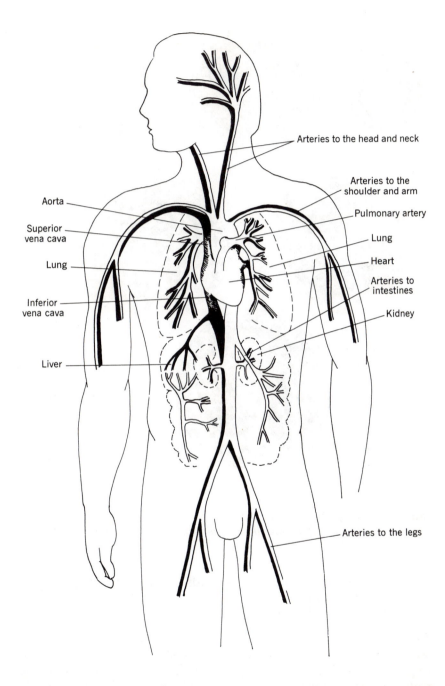

Arteries to the head and neck

Arteries to the shoulder and arm

Pulmonary artery

Aorta

Superior vena cava

Lung

Lung

Heart

Inferior vena cava

Arteries to intestines

Kidney

Liver

Arteries to the legs

Figure 5.1   *Human circulatory system, showing principal arteries and veins.*

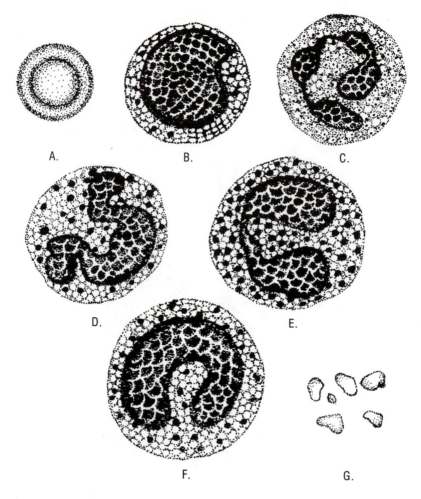

Figure 5.2   *Human blood cells. (A) Erythrocyte (red blood cell); (B) lympho-cyte; (C) neutrophil; (D) basophil; (E) eosinophil; (F) monocyte; (G) platelets (fragments of cells).*

carbohydrates (mainly sugars), fats (lipids), minerals, waste products, hormones, and dissolved gases. As already indicated, red blood cells and white blood cells are suspended in the plasma.

RED BLOOD CELLS

RBCs are tiny, disk-shaped cells. Their main function is to carry oxygen from the lungs to the tissues. This ability to carry oxygen is made possible by the component *hemoglobin,* which is also responsible for the red color of these cells. The more oxygen present, the brighter red their color. Red blood cells are by far the most numerous cells in the blood; they average from 4.5 to 5 million per cubic millimeter of blood.

WHITE BLOOD CELLS

WBCs consist of various types of colorless cells. They can change their shape, leave the blood vessels, and move between the cells of the body. These properties help the WBCs to destroy disease-causing organisms (pathogens). Attracted to any area of tissue in which pathogens are present, such as the site of a wound or infection, WBCs engulf (or ingest) the pathogens and destroy them. Often, however, WBCs are killed by the poisons (toxins) given off by these pathogens and become part of the accumulation of material known as *pus*. Far less numerous than RBCs, there are about 7,000 WBCs per cubic millimeter of blood in an adult.

PLATELETS

Platelets are microscopic fragments of larger cells. Also known as *thrombocytes* (Figure 5.2), they are essential to the process of blood clotting, or *coagulation*. When a blood vessel is damaged, platelets release *thromboplastin* (which may also be released by damaged tissues). This reacts in stages with two plasma proteins, *prothrombin* and *fibrinogen,* to form a meshwork of *fibrin threads* that entrap blood cells, thus forming a clot. Fibrin threads are sticky and adhere easily to any blood vessel opening. Platelets normally number 150,000 to 300,000 per cubic millimeter of blood.

Blood Groups

As a result of severe blood loss or other reasons, it is sometimes necessary to transfuse *whole blood* into a person. Although substitutes such as plasma may be used, nothing takes the place of whole blood. Not all blood is alike, however, and blood cannot be transfused into a person carelessly. The mixing of some blood types causes the blood to clump, or *agglutinate,* when antigens in donor blood combine with antibodies of recipient blood.

Blood is typed on the basis of the antigens present in its red blood cells. While every person actually has *many* blood types (antigens in the RBCs), there are only two blood-group series that are of consequence in most transfusions, the A-B-O series and the Rh series. A few people, however, carry high antibody levels against antigens in other blood-group series (such as the M-N series), further complicating transfusion for these people. Even though the A-B-O and Rh groupings for a unit of whole blood are appropriate for the recipient, the blood must still be cross-matched on a slide with a drop of the recipient's blood to detect any possible agglutination. Such agglutination might result in the breakdown (hemolysis) of red blood cells, circulatory shock, kidney failure, or death.

Anemias

Although the word *"anemia"* literally means "lack of blood," it is actually used to describe any condition in which the oxygen-carrying capacity of the blood is reduced. Anemia can result from a variety of conditions, including loss of blood (hemorrhage), deficient red cell production, excessive red cell destruction, nutritional inadequacies, or genetic disorders.

NUTRITIONAL ANEMIAS

The most common anemia, *deficiency anemia,* is the result of an iron-deficient diet and is most frequently seen in females. This type of anemia can be corrected with proper diet planning or with the use of iron supplements in pill or liquid form. Occasionally iron injections are given when the deficiency is severe.

Another important nutritional anemia, *pernicious anemia,* is associated with a lack of vitamin B_{12} (cobalamine). Cobalamine functions as a coenzyme in the formation of red blood cells. B_{12} is usually present in the dirt, but the intestines of some people lack a substance necessary for its absorption into the blood. The tendency toward this problem is hereditary. In pernicious anemia, the red cells are characteristically larger and have less pigment (hemoglobin) than normal red cells. Their oxygen-carrying capacity is severely decreased. Without injections of B_{12}, death is the eventual outcome.

APLASTIC ANEMIA

Aplastic anemia is associated with impairment of the blood-forming functions of the bone marrow. It is most common in adolescents and young adults. While aplastic anemia is sometimes a result of chromosomal defects, it is usually the result of ingesting a toxic chemical agent. The bone marrow produces a deficient number of red cells, and these cells exhibit atypical structural formations. The general symptoms are severe, including waxy pallor of the skin and multiple internal hemorrhages throughout the body. Administration of whole blood transfusions is the main therapy.

SICKLE CELL ANEMIA

A hereditary type of anemia of special importance to black people is *sickle cell anemia.* In this disorder, a minor chemical abnormality in the hemoglobin of the red blood cells causes them to appear elongated and sometimes sickle-shaped, instead of the normal round shape (Figure 5.3). Since sickled cells tend to flow through the smaller blood vessels with more friction, they bunch up in some of the tiny capillaries so that blood clots form. Typically, symptoms begin to appear between the ages of 2 and 4 years, including weakness, poor

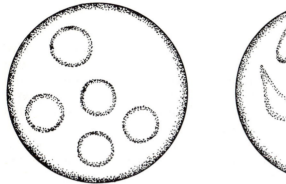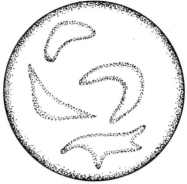

Fig. 5.3 *Sickle cell anemia. Left, normal red blood cells; right, sickled cells.*

appetite, frequent illnesses and infections, pain in the joints and elsewhere, sores on the ankles, and anemia. The most characteristic symptom of the disease is the "sickle cell crisis," during which there is high fever, excruciating pain, and the possibility of death from blood clots forming in the lungs, kidneys, or brain.

A child may inherit the recessive gene for sickle cell from one or both parents; the difference between a single dose and a double dose of sickle cell means the difference between health and disease. Someone who has inherited the trait from only one of his parents is called a "carrier." He will not have sickle cell anemia himself, but he will carry a gene for the disease in his cells and may pass it on to his children.

About 1 in 10 black Americans is a carrier of sickle cell disease; about 1 in 100 black couples are *both* carriers, and they risk a 1 in 4 chance of having a child with sickle cell anemia each time a pregnancy occurs. Thus, about 1 in 400 black babies born in this country has sickle cell anemia. Currently, about half of these people die before age 20, though improved treatment methods are extending the lives of sickle cell anemia victims.

Sickle cell disease also occurs among black peoples of Africa, the Caribbean, Latin America, and Southern India, and it occurs occasionally among whites of Mediterranean origin.

Considerable research is taking place on treatments for sickle cell anemia but a real cure remains to be developed. However, several simple and inexpensive tests are available for detecting individuals who are carriers of the gene. They can then be counseled on the advisability of selecting mates who are not also carriers of the gene or on the risk of sickle cell anemia among any children they might produce.

The Heart

Structure of the Heart

Approximately the size of a fist and weighing about three-quarters of a pound, the heart is a mass of cardiac muscle richly interwoven with blood vessels. It is centrally located between the lungs, a bit to the left of the midline of the body. Shaped like a cone, its tip (apex) is directed downward and to the left. The heart is actually a double pump with a central wall, or *septum,* separating the right and left sides (Figure 5.4). There are two chambers on each side. The two upper chambers are called the *atria,* the lower two chambers the *ventricles.* Each chamber has a specific name: the *right atrium,* the *right ventricle,* the *left atrium,* and the *left ventricle.* The atria are "receiving chambers"; the ventricles are "pumping chambers" and thus are larger and have thicker muscular walls.

The muscular wall of the heart is the *myocardium.* Its inner surface is covered with a thin lining called the *endocardium;* its outer surface is covered with a thin membrane called the *epicardium.* The heart is enclosed in a saclike *pericardium* in which there is a small

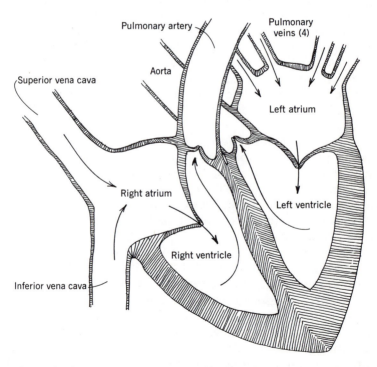

Figure 5.4 *The four chambers of the heart and valves that guard their openings, as seen from the front. Arrows indicate the direction of blood flow.*

amount of fluid to lubricate the outer surface of the heart in its movements.

Each side of the heart represents an independent pump. The right atrium receives *deoxygenated* (oxygen-deficient) blood from all parts of the body by way of the network of veins. The veins above the heart merge to become the *superior vena cava;* those below merge to become the *inferior vena cava.* The two venae cavae carry blood into the right atrium, which then pumps the blood past the *tricuspid valve* into the right ventricle. When the right ventricle contracts, blood cannot pass backward through the now closed valve, which allows blood to flow in only one direction. Instead the blood is pumped out past the *pulmonary semilunar valve* into the *pulmonary artery,* which carries the blood to the lungs. The function of the pulmonary semilunar valve is to prevent blood from flowing back into the right ventricle. In the lungs the blood is *oxygenated* (gets rid of much of its carbon dioxide and receives oxygen).

Following oxygenation, the blood returns to the left side of the heart by way of the *pulmonary veins,* which empty into the left atrium. Upon contraction, the left atrium pumps the blood past the *bicuspid (mitral) valve* into the left ventricle. The left ventricle pumps the blood past the *aortic semilunar valve* into the *aorta,* the largest artery of the body. The two valves on the left side of the heart serve the same function as those on the right (Figure 5.5).

The tricuspid and bicuspid valves are both called *atrioventricular valves* since they are located between the atrium and ventricle on each respective side. To prevent these valves from collapsing when the ventricles contract, strong cords (*chordae tendineae*) attach to the leaflets of the valves and anchor them to the papillary muscles in the wall of each ventricle (Figure 5.4 and 5.5).

Heart Action

The heart muscle operates unlike any other muscle of the body. Although the heart is under the control and regulation of the brain, its beat originates independently in the heart muscle itself. The beat starts in the wall of the right atrium at a spot called the *sinoatrial node (SA node or pacemaker),* as shown in Figure 5.6. This node consists of a small mass of specialized cardiac muscle. From it an impulse travels over the entire atrial muscle, causing both atria to contract simultaneously and forcing the blood down into both ventricles at the same instant. The impulse is then passed to a second specialized area, the *atrioventricular node (AV node),* located between the right atrium and the ventricles (Figure 5.6). From this spot the impulse is transmitted to the *bundle of His* (a band of specialized muscle cells in the septum between the ventricles) and to fibers that spread out from

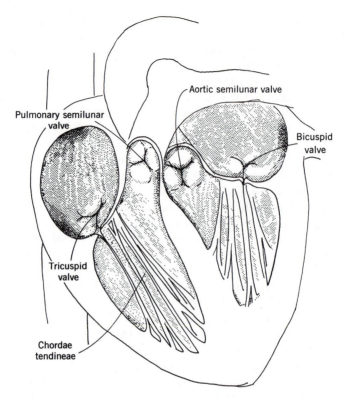

Figure 5.5.   *The four valves of the heart and the chordae tendineae, as seen from the front.*

the apex of the heart up through both ventricular walls. Thus, upon impulse, the muscles of both ventricles contract simultaneously, forcing the blood upward into the pulmonary artery and aorta, respectively. Any degeneration of the AV node or bundle of His results in a *heart block*.

In the normal heartbeat, the two atria contract at the same time, while the ventricles relax. When the ventricles contract, the atria relax. The phase of contraction is called *systole,* and the phase of relaxation is called *diastole*. Following ventricular systole, the entire heart pauses momentarily.

HEARTBEAT

The heartbeat rate of a person at rest averages between 70 and 75 beats per minute. Following athletic training, the normal heart rate decreases, occasionally to as low as 45 beats per minute. The heart compensates for this by pumping more blood each beat. The heart rate in a person who is not in good physical condition may be as high

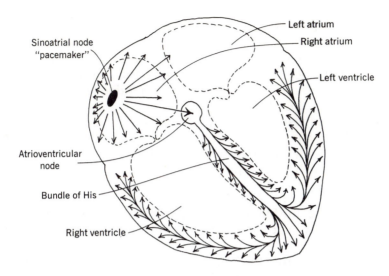

Figure 5.6 *Transmission of the heart impulse from the sinoatrial node to the atrioventricular node and then throughout the walls of the ventricles.*

as 90 to 100 beats per minute. Such an ill-conditioned heart also pumps less blood each beat. It is less strenuous for the heart to beat fewer times per minute, since this causes less heart fatigue and gives the heart more time to relax.

HEART OUTPUT

The adult heart pumps about 5 quarts of blood per minute. The amount of blood pumped with each beat (*cardiac output*) does not necessarily relate to the rate of heartbeat. As we have just seen, some individuals have a higher rate of heartbeat, but pump less blood with each beat. This may happen when the heart muscle becomes defective. Cardiac output is affected by exercise, large meals, pregnancy, sleep, and emotional stresses. Heart attacks may occur following overeating or emotional outbursts. This is more likely if the heart is already defective and has insufficient reserve power to match the added oxygen demands of the body.

BLOOD PRESSURE

With each beat of the heart, blood is forced out of the left ventricle into the arteries. Since the arteries are small and have elastic walls, pressure is required to force the blood through these vessels. The blood is always under some pressure. The *systolic pressure* caused by the contraction of the left ventricle is greatest; the *diastolic pressure* between contractions is least.

Blood pressure is measured as systolic pressure over diastolic pressure, which averages 120 millimeters over 80 millimeters of mercury (how high the pressure will push a column of mercury). Blood pressure may be modified by such things as blood "thickness" (viscosity), elasticity of the arteries, cardiac output, obstructions at the valves or in the arteries, and age. Arteries tend to lose their elasticity with age, and this results in a corresponding increase in systolic pressure. The most desirable blood pressure for a given individual is sufficient blood pressure to maintain proper circulation to all parts of the body, but not such excessive pressure that the arteries may burst, causing hemorrhage and possible death.

PULSE

The pulsation of the blood through the arteries as a result of ventricular contraction can be easily felt wherever an artery is near the surface of the skin. The *pulse* is the result of pressure on the walls of the arteries. Starting from the heart, a wave of pressure moves down the arteries with each heartbeat. This is not an indication of the speed of blood movement in the arteries. (The speed of blood movement decreases the farther the blood travels.) The number of pulsations each minute, or the *pulse rate,* is the same as the heart rate. The pulse is commonly counted on the inside of the wrist, the side of the throat, or over the temples.

Blood Vessels

The vessels that carry blood away from the heart are called *arteries,* while those that carry blood toward the heart are called *veins.* The arteries have relatively thicker and stronger walls than the veins. Artery walls consist of three layers. The middle layer is made up of elastic and smooth muscle fibers. These muscles not only allow the arteries to stretch with increased blood pressure, which we recognize as pulse, but constrict upon nerve impulse to narrow the internal size of the artery.

The smallest subdivisions of the arteries are called *arterioles,* which lead into the smallest vessels of the body, the *capillaries.* The capillaries serve as a connecting link between the arterioles and *venules* (the smallest veins of the body). Microscopic in size, the capillaries form extensive networks through the various body tissues. Their walls are very thin, usually only one cell layer. Because of their small size and thin walls, the capillaries afford the blood close contact with the vessel walls, allowing rapid diffusion to occur. This diffusion is aided by the very slow movement of the blood through the capillaries. After passing through the capillaries the blood is collected in the venules.

The venules unite to form small veins that combine to form larger veins which return the blood to the heart. Compared with arteries, the veins have thinner walls and less muscle and elastic tissue. Some of the veins in the limbs are even provided with valves to prevent the blood from flowing backward into the capillaries.

The blood vessels carrying blood from the right ventricle to the lungs and back to the heart are responsible for *pulmonary circulation*. Vessels transporting the blood from the left ventricle to all parts of the body and back to the right atrium are responsible for *systemic circulation*. These coronary vessels leave the aorta through two small arteries just above the aortic semilunar valve, flow over the surface of the heart, and return their blood to the right atrium.

Lymphatics

The materials that escape from the blood in the capillaries enter the intercellular tissue fluid known as *lymph*. Lymph accumulates between the cells faster than it is able to move back into the blood capillaries. As a result, it must be continually drained from the tissue space through a system of vessels called the *lymphatic system* (Figure 5.7). Completely separate from the blood capillaries, these lymph vessels begin as microscopic, blind (closed) ducts in all parts of the body. Branches of lymphatic vessels unite as they converge into the *thoracic duct* and the *right lymphatic duct*, which eventually enter the veins of the neck.

The thin-walled lymphatic vessels are provided with valves to prevent backflow. Exercise and changes in body position help these valves to maintain the flow of lymph. The lymphatic system has no pump, or heart, with which to push the lymph along.

As the lymph passes to the veins of the neck, it moves through a series of filters called *lymph nodes* (lymph glands). These nodes remove and tend to destroy impurities such as cancer cells, dead blood cells, and pathogens. These foreign particles and bacteria are then ingested and partly destroyed by certain white blood cells normally present in the nodes. The nodes also manufacture some of the white blood cells and produce antibodies.

Lymph nodes close to cancer sites tend to collect wandering cancer cells. Thus these nodes are commonly surgically removed along with the cancerous tissue.

Types and Causes of Circulatory Diseases

Congenital Disorders

Congenital defects are those which are present at the time of birth. Most congenital heart defects arise during the first three months of fetal development. Although the specific causes of many congenital defects are unknown, some of the known causes include diseases, such as German measles; drugs; and exposure to X rays or other radiation.

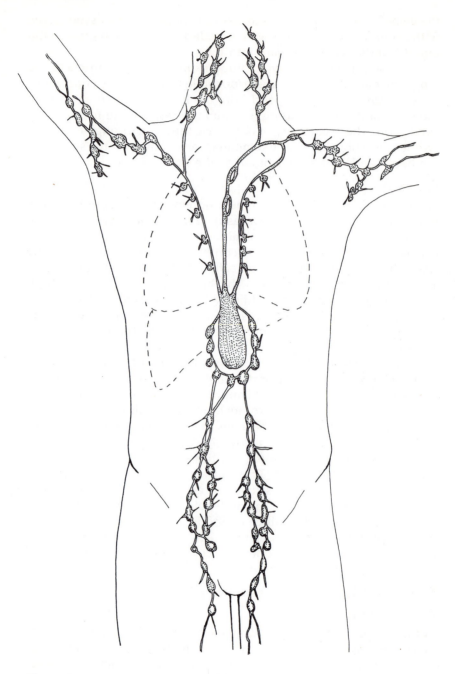

Figure 5.7   *Lymphatic system of the body.*

Heart malformations are common in all parts of the world. Most of them present severe handicaps to children. Such inborn heart defects are thought to be due to developmental accidents, not to inheritance. A mother with a congenital heart defect has only about a 2-percent-above-average chance of passing such a malformity on to her children.

KINDS OF CONGENITAL HEART DEFECTS

Defects may affect any part of the heart. The extent of the malformation may be slight or extensive. Because some defects cause reduction in the normal supply of oxygenated blood, the skin takes on a bluish hue. Consequently, a newborn showing such a condition generally is called a "blue baby." Some of the more common forms of congential heart defects are outlined in Table 5.1 (pages 92–94).

RESEARCH AND REPAIR OF CONGENITAL DEFECTS

Until about 30 years ago only about 1 of every 3 congenital heart victims survived to the age of 10. However, through the development of the *heart-lung machine,* a device that takes over the functions of the heart and lungs while they are bypassed for surgical repair, open-heart surgery is now possible. Such surgery may involve closing holes, repairing or replacing defective valves, or repairing other defects. The heart-lung machine is also used in operations for the repair of major arteries and veins, heart transplants, and the implantation of devices into the heart. Although improvements are being made in the repair of congenital heart defects, the ultimate goal of cardiology is to discover what causes these defects and to find ways of preventing them.

Degenerative Cardiovascular Disorders

Although the heart is resistant to disorders, many things can reduce its efficiency. Heart disease may be the result of infections, toxins (poisons), injuries, poor nutrition, inactivity, or other disturbances that weaken the heart. Diseases of the heart and blood vessels, the *cardiovascular diseases,* are the leading cause of death in this country. The major cardiovascular diseases are described below.

RHEUMATIC HEART DISEASE

Much heart disease in childhood is the result of *rheumatic fever,* which usually first attacks the individual between the ages of 5 and 15.

A small percentage of persons suffering from streptococcal infections develop the symptoms of rheumatic fever (swelling and pain in the joints, accompanied by fever). The original infection may be in any part of the body, but it will likely be strep throat, scarlet fever, or middle-ear infection. Rheumatic fever is actually an allergic response to a streptococcal infection, in which the antibodies produced

TABLE 5.1   Congenital Heart and Circulatory Defects

Congenital Malformations	Definition or Explanation of Malformation
Tetralogy of fallot	A malformation of the heart involving four distinct defects: 1. An opening in the wall between the lower chambers of the heart (ventricular septal defect). 2. Misplacement of the aorta, "overriding" the abnormal opening, so that it receives blood from both the right and left lower chambers instead of only the left. 3. Narrowing of the pulmonary valve (pulmonic stenosis). 4. Enlargement of the right lower chamber of the heart (hypertrophy of right ventricle).
Interventricular septal defect	An opening in the wall (septum) between the right and left ventricles permitting passage of blood between the two ventricles.
Interatrial septal defect	An opening in the wall (septum) between the right and left atria permitting passage of blood between the two atria.

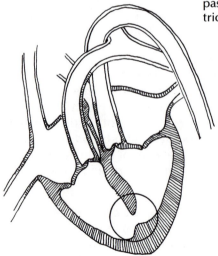

TABLE 5.1 (Continued) Congenital Heart and Circulatory Defects

Congenital Malformations	*Definition or Explanation of Malformation*
Patent ductus arteriosus 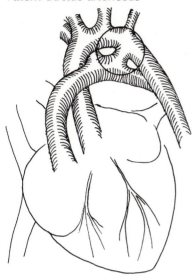	A defect in which a small duct between the aorta and the pulmonary artery, which normally closes soon after birth, remains open. As a result, blood from both sides of the heart is pumped into the pulmonary artery and into the lungs.
Patent foramen ovale 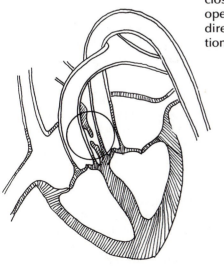	A defect in which an oval hole between the left and right upper chambers (atria) of the heart, which normally closes shortly after birth, remains open. This allows the passage of blood directly from venous to arterial circulation without going through the lungs.

TABLE 5.1   (Continued) Congenital Heart and Circulatory Defects

Congenital Malformations	*Definition or Explanation of Malformation*
Coarctation (of aorta) 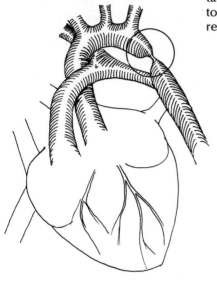	Literally, "pressing together." A congenital defect in which there is a pressing together or narrowing of the aorta that restricts the flow of blood.
Transposition of great vessels	A condition in which the pulmonary artery arises from the left ventricle while the aorta arises from the right ventricle. (These vessels would normally connect to the opposite ventricles.)
Eisenmenger complex	A combination of ventricular septal defects, right ventricular hypertrophy, and an aorta connected with the right ventricle.
Fibroelastosis cordis	A condition in which the lining of the left ventricle (endocardium) is coverted into a thick fibroelastic layer with a reduction in the blood-holding capacity of the ventricle.

against the bacteria attack certain of the person's own tissues. In about 60 percent of the cases the heart is inflamed, and in about 25 percent of the cases it may be permanently damaged.

Although other layers of the heart may be infected, the most common damage is done to the endocardium (the inner lining of the heart). Inflammation of the endocardium (*endocarditis*) causes the heart valves, which consist primarily of endocardium, to become scarred. (The bicuspid valve is particularly susceptible to scarring.) Blood deposits on such scarred valves; they thicken and either lose their flexibility or stick together. Thus they are prevented from opening or closing completely. The blood may leak back through the valve, forcing the heart to pump harder in order to circulate an adequate supply of blood.

Open-heart surgery has been increasingly effective in relieving such damage. The scar tissue may be removed, or the damaged valves may be replaced with artificial valves (Figure 5.8).

Antibiotics have lowered the incidence of and death rate from rheumatic fever. As a preventive measure, all streptococcal infections should be promptly brought to the attention of a physician. A person with a history of rheumatic fever must be particularly prompt in seeking treatment for infections, as one attack leaves him highly susceptible to repeated attacks.

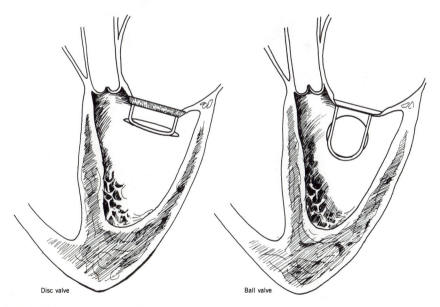

Disc valve   Ball valve

Figure 5.8 *Two types of commonly used artificial heart valves. These valves have replaced diseased bicuspid valves.*

HEART MURMURS

Heart murmurs are abnormal sounds produced by vibrations that result from improperly working heart valves. They may be due to the endocarditis of rheumatic fever. The murmur heard through a stethoscope results from an incompletely closing valve so that blood flows back across a valve into a heart chamber as it relaxes, causing a swishing sound.

Murmurs are occasionally heard in hearts that are actually normal. A young person may engage in such strenuous exercise that the flow of blood through the valves creates a temporary turbulence or murmur.

ATHEROSCLEROSIS

Atherosclerosis, one of the most important circulatory problems in the United States today, is a disease of the arteries. Cholesterol and other lipids (fatty materials) deposit in the walls of the arteries, narrowing the diameter of the channel *(lumen)* of the artery and causing roughness of the inner lining (Figure 5.9). Among the results are

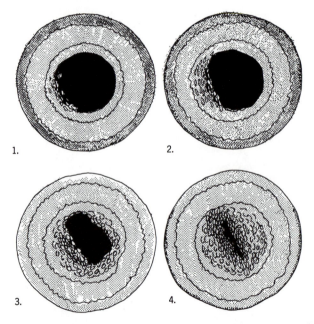

Figure 5.9 *The closure effects of atherosclerosis within an artery. (1) Plaques of cholesterol invade the tunica intima. As more cholesterol is laid down (2 and 3), the inner wall protrudes into the channel, or lumen, of the artery. In time the lumen becomes severely obstructed (4) and will eventually close as a result of the effects of cholesterol or the formation of a clot in the diseased artery.*

reduced circulation of blood, increased blood pressure, and the formation of blood clots (*thrombi*) in the damaged arteries.

More specifically, when atherosclerosis narrows the coronary arteries supplying the heart muscle, the results may include *angina pectoris* (pains in the chest, indicating inadequate oxygen supply to the heart muscle) or *coronary thrombosis* (formation of a blood clot in a coronary artery, the most common form of *heart attack*).

Similarly, when atherosclerosis affects the arteries supplying the brain the results may include *senility*, the mental deterioration of an elderly person (atherosclerosis is not the only cause), or *strokes*, when blood clots block the arteries serving the brain.

Other problem areas include the legs and feet, where atherosclerosis may lead to gangrene, and the kidneys, resulting in high blood pressure. While the consequences of atherosclerosis usually appear in older persons, there is evidence that the process leading to these problems often begins in youth.

While the causes of atherosclerosis are still not definitely known, several factors have been associated with the process. Among possible dietary causes are high cholesterol intake, high consumption of animal fats, and the presence of large amounts of table sugar (sucrose) in the diet. Each of these factors has some scientific support and all may be important. Among nondietary factors, emotional stress and lack of exercise have both been implicated as causes of atherosclerosis.

HYPERTENSION

Hypertension is high blood pressure, a common problem in the United States. The incidence of hypertension increases with age, though it does occur among younger people as well. The incidence is also higher among blacks than among whites and among females than among males (Table 5.2). Many deaths are a direct result of hypertension.

In many cases no cause for hypertension is apparent. These cases are known as *essential hypertension,* probably a hereditary condition. Among the many known causes of hypertension are emotional

TABLE 5.2 Incidence of Hypertension

Age Group	Males		Females	
	Black	*White*	*Black*	*White*
45–64	37.2%	18.1%	40.2%	21.5%
65–79	54.2%	26.1%	65.3%	46.1%

Source. "Health in the Later Years of Life," U.S. Department of Health, Education, and Welfare, Public Health Service, October 1971.

stress, obesity, kidney disease, hardening of the arteries, hormonal disorders, and excessive salt in the diet. The treatment of hypertension may involve low-sodium diets, weight control, resolution of emotional problems, and various medications.

Hypertension is damaging for two reasons: (1) It puts an excess work load on the heart and the left ventricle in particular. (2) The arteries may be damaged by excessive pressure. A hypertensive patient tends to develop cardiovascular ailments much sooner than a person not suffering from hypertension. The high blood pressure in the arteries causes a "hardening" (*sclerosis*) of blood vessels all over the body. The vessels become weakened; clots tend to form in them much more easily; some vessels rupture and hemorrhage. Hemorrhages in the vessels of the brain (*cerebral hemorrhages*) and vessels of the kidneys are particulary destructive.

CEREBROVASCULAR ACCIDENTS (STROKES)

The brain receives over one-fifth of all the blood pumped by the heart. Since the neurons (nerve cells) are extremely sensitive to any oxygen shortage, dying within a few minutes, any interruption in the normal flow of blood to the brain may have serious consequences. Such interruptions, usually called "strokes," may occur in several ways, as shown in Table 5.3. Most strokes result from rupture of vessels (hemorrhages) or from blood clots forming in the vessels.

Depending on the size and location of the affected area of the brain, the results of a stroke range from minor damage to rapid death. Typical results of moderate-size strokes include speech impediments, some degree of paralysis (often one-sided), loss of memory or other mental function, and blindness.

Considerable progress has been made in both the treatment and rehabilitation of stroke patients. While some individuals lead a restricted life because of the permanent loss of some brain function, many others recover completely from strokes.

VARICOSE VEINS

In the discussion of veins, it was mentioned that some of the veins of the body, such as those in the legs, are provided with valves to prevent the backflow of blood as it is raised to the heart. These valves may be destroyed when veins are overstretched by an excess amount of blood for a prolonged period of time. (See Figure 5.10.) This sometimes occurs in pregnancy or when a person stands much of the time. Stretched veins become larger in cross section, but the valves do not stretch accordingly. Thus the valves fail to prevent the backflow of blood. The result is increased blood pressure in these veins. Eventually, the valves stop functioning entirely. Such large, protruding veins beneath the skin in the feet, legs, or female genitalia are

TABLE 5.3   Ways in Which Strokes Occur

Cause	*Explanation*
Hemorrhage (bleeding) 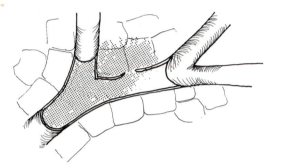	The wall of an artery of the brain breaks, permitting blood to escape and thus damage surrounding brain tissue; such escape reduces the flow of blood to other brain parts.
Thrombosis (clot formation) 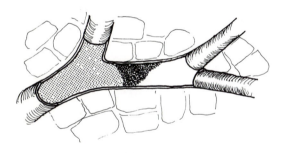	A clot of blood forms in an artery of the brain and stops the flow of blood to the part of the brain supplied by the clot-plugged artery.
Embolism (blocking of a vessel by a clot floating in the bloodstream) 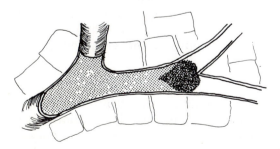	A clot from a diseased blood vessel is pumped to the brain and stops up one of the brain's arteries.

TABLE 5.3   (Continued)   Ways in Which Strokes Occur

Cause	Explanation
Compression (pressure)	A tumor, swollen brain tissue, or a large clot from another vessel presses upon a vessel of the brain and stops its flow of blood.

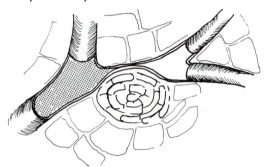

Cause	Explanation
Spasm (tightening and closing down of walls of an artery)	An artery of the brain constricts and thus reduces the flow of blood to an area of the brain. If the spasm is of short duration permanent damage may not occur.

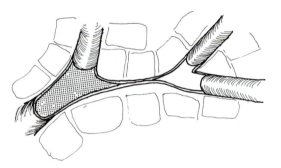

called *varicose veins.* Circulation in surrounding muscles is inadequate, and nutrients fail to diffuse into such tissues properly. Muscles often become painful and weak, and the skin may become ulcerated.

Therapy for varicose veins includes elevating the legs to heart level or binding them tightly. The legs may also be injected with certain agents that harden and plug the most protruding veins. The weakened sections of veins may even be removed surgically; the blood is then carried by other veins.

SHOCK

Circulatory shock is a progressive condition caused by reduced blood flow. Since the brain is deprived of an adequate blood supply, shock may rapidly kill a person. Many conditions can lead to circulatory shock. It can result from a loss of blood or a reduced heart output. The cause can also be an emotional reaction. In this type of shock

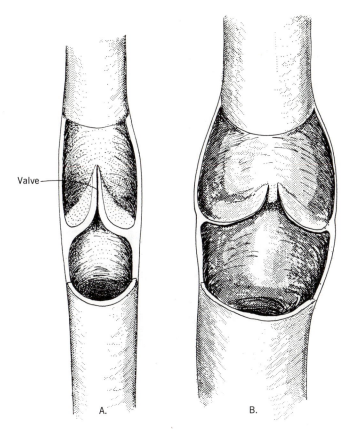

Valve

Figure 5.10 *Venous valves. (A) The vein enlarges as its walls weaken. (B) The valves give way and the vein walls distend as blood reservoirs at the site. Such vein protrudings are visible on the surface of the skin as varicose veins.*

(called *neurogenic shock*), the blood vessels lose their muscle tone, dilate, and allow blood to pool in the systemic circulation.

The symptoms of circulatory shock include mental haziness, dizziness, and fainting. Any person who shows signs of shock or who faints should be kept lying completely horizontal, with his head level. If this does not relieve the symptoms promptly, the person should receive immediate medical attention.

Coronary Heart Disease

The coronary blood vessels surrounding the heart derive their name from the fact that they encircle the heart like a crown or corona. (See Figure 5.11.) These vessels transport almost a half pint of blood every minute to the heart muscle. Any sudden blockage of one of the coronary arteries deprives a section of the heart of its blood supply;

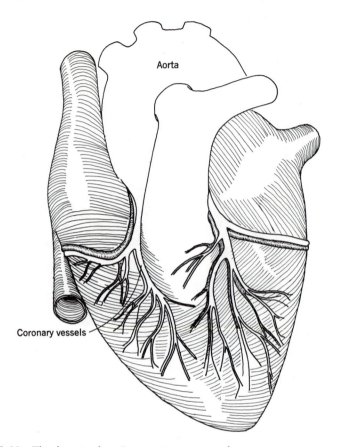

Figure 5.11   *The heart, showing coronary vessels.*

cardiac cells die, heart contractions may cease, and circulation may come to a standstill. If a coronary artery is completely plugged, the condition is called a *coronary occlusion* or *heart attack*. If the obstruction is only partial or is in one of the smaller coronary tributaries, prompt treatment often leads to the individual's recovery. An occlusion in a main coronary artery is very serious and may cause sudden death. Causes of coronary disease include atherosclerosis, aging, emotional stress, obesity, smoking, and hypertension.

Pain from the heart may be due to a blood-flow deficiency in the coronary vessels. This may be referred to (actually felt in) the left arm and shoulder. Such pain from the heart is called *angina pectoris* (chest pain). Angina pectoris may not actually be noticed until the work load is too great in relation to the blood flow in the coronary vessels. Some people do not feel pain unless they exercise or experience strong emotion; others experience it much of the time.

Fortunately, the great majority of coronary disease patients recover and are able to lead active, useful lives, providing they receive proper treatment under good medical supervision. Approximately one-fourth of all deaths in the United States, however, still result from coronary artery diseases. Also, it is estimated that more than 1 out of every 10 Americans suffers some degree of insufficiency of blood supply to the heart.

FACTORS RELATING TO HEART DISEASE

Any difference in the frequency and distribution of coronary artery disease should be explainable by differences in people's heredity, environment, nutrition, or habits. Heart research has been unable either to place these factors in order of importance or to show that any one of them is decisive. Nevertheless, evidence that these factors are all related to cardiovascular diseases is accumulating. Studies have made it possible to pick out individuals who are high risks for heart disease. Table 5.4 lists the factors that tend to pinpoint individuals who are likely to have a heart attack.

SYMPTOMS OF CORONARY HEART DISEASE

Some types of coronary heart disease are symptomless. When symptoms are present, they can sometimes be mistaken for those of other body disorders. For example, dizziness is common to many disorders. Legitimate symptoms of coronary heart disease are often overlooked. Breathlessness, for example, may be mistakenly attributed to bronchitis, or coughing to smoking. Generally, however, there are certain important symptoms that should be looked for and referred to a physician. These are explained in Table 5.5.

TREATMENT OF HEART DISEASE

The treatment selected for a heart patient depends on the nature of his disease and how critical his case is. A chronic illness (one slowly affecting the individual) usually permits time for more deliberate diagnosis and treatment. Surgery for the repair of congenital conditions, for example, may be planned some time in advance. In a critical, sudden heart attack, however, prompt diagnosis and treatment are needed.

EMERGENCY CARE   The person who has just had a heart attack is in need of immediate emergency care and should be taken to a hospital at once. The first medical treatment is usually to provide the oxygen that the weakened heart is unable to supply. This may involve the use of oxygen, drugs (such as nitroglycerin) to dilate the obstructed blood vessels, or electric or drug stimulators to revive the faltering heart. Next, measurements are needed for pulse and blood pressure, electrocardiograms to record the electric impulses of the heart, or

TABLE 5.4 Factors Relating to Heart Disease

Factor	Explanation	Risk Involved
Serum cholesterol	Refers to cholesterol carried in liquid portion of blood. The amount of cholesterol in the blood is believed to relate to diet.	A person with serum cholesterol over 240 mg. % has more than three times the risk of a person with less than 200 mg. %.
Age		A male in his 50s has four times the risk of attack as one in his 30s.
Blood pressure	Refers to elevated levels of blood pressure, or hypertension.	A person with systolic blood pressure greater than 160 has four times the risk of attack as one with SBP of less than 120.
Cigarette smoking	Refers to any cigarette smoker, although the greater the amount and the longer the smoking history, the greater the risk. Pipe and cigar smoking do not appear related.	A cigarette smoker has nearly twice the risk of attack as a nonsmoker.
Vital capacity	Refers to amount of air a person can forcefully inhale and exhale.	An individual with low vital capacity has about twice the risk of attack as an individual with high vital capacity.
EKG abnormalities	Refers to recording of electrical activity related to the contraction of cardiac muscle.	An individual with an EKG abnormality has 2½ times the risk of an individual with normal EKG.
Miscellaneous suspected factors: Gross obesity Insufficient physical activity Inheritance		

Source: The Framingham Heart Study, National Heart Institute, Public Health Service, U. S. Dept. Health, Education, and Welfare.

TABLE 5.5   Possible Symptoms of Heart Disease

Symptom

Breathlessness	Unusual shortness of breath associated with moderate exertion might be an early symptom of a weakened heart muscle. It signals a marked oxygen shortage somewhere in the body. If, for instance, a person is out of breath after climbing one flight of stairs, he should see his physician.
Chest pains	Pain or a tight feeling in the chest during or after exertion or excitement may be due to oxygen deficiency. Cardiac pain is often in the center of the chest, very pressing, and may move to the shoulders and arms. Chest pains may also result from other causes, but it is best to be safe and consult a physician when such pains occur.
Swelling of feet and ankles	If the heart fails to pump with usual vigor, the blood flow slows down and fluid may gather in the tissues (*edema*). This may be noticed first in the feet and ankles. It also may occur from other causes.
Persistent fatigue	Frequent tiredness without apparent reason may be a sign of heart difficulty or hypertension. Other possible symptoms of heart disease may include a heavy feeling in the limbs, weakness, and lack of vigor during or following exertion.
Miscellaneous symptoms	Other symptoms that may occur in some cardiac patients include *cyanosis* (blueness of skin due to insufficient oxygen in blood), loss of consciousness, recurrent bronchitis, and heart palpitations.

X-ray and fluoroscopic examinations to measure the size and outline of the heart. All efforts must be made as soon as possible to reduce the blood-pumping load placed on the heart by reducing the patient's physical exertion and emotional excitement.

The first week (and especially the first 48 hours) after a heart attack is the most critical period. The largest number of deaths from heart attacks occur during this time. The danger of death is reduced as time goes on. With coronary patients, new blood vessels gradually form around the obstructed vessels, setting up new circulation, and an adequate oxygen-food supply is slowly restored to the deprived cells. Scar tissue forms over the affected area, and slowly, as the heart returns to normal, the patient can resume many normal activities.

LONG-TERM CARE   The cardinal rule of all treatment for heart patients is to prevent anginal discomfort (pain brought on by an inadequate oxygen supply to the heart). Absence of such pain is a good indication that the heart muscle is receiving adequate circulation. To help circulation, drugs are often used: digitalis for a fuller heartbeat; nitrates, such as nitroglycerin, to dilate coronary blood vessels and reduce pressure; anticoagulants to reduce the possibility of clotting; sedative drugs to quiet the body; and other drugs to cause certain actions to take place in the kidneys to help relieve pressure in the heart. A diet is set up which includes all essential foods in adequate amounts. The person must learn to rest and limit activity. Schedules of moderate exercises must be established. Physicians usually insist that their patients lose any excess weight and stop smoking.

Bypass surgery has emerged in recent years as an important but controversial treatment for severe coronary artery disease. This surgery involves removing a section of blood vessel from elsewhere in the body, such as the thigh, and using it to carry additional blood to the heart muscle. The diseased section of coronary artery is thus bypassed. Through this procedure, many persons who might otherwise have died or been severely restricted in their activities have been restored to good health and full activity. Others have died during or within a few months following surgery, but many of these people would have died anyway. In any case, candidates for bypass surgery are carefully selected.

Prevention of Cardiovascular Diseases

Whether or not cardiovascular disorders are preventable largely depends upon their causes. Diseases due to infection or malnutrition are often preventable. Heart damage caused by rheumatic fever can be prevented by reducing the incidence and severity of rheumatic fever with prompt use of antibiotics in treating streptococcal infections. On the other hand, it is impossible to predict or prevent many of the congenital malformations of the heart and blood vessels.

Circulatory problems can be greatly reduced by a reduction in cigarette smoking. The prevention of atherosclerosis appears to depend upon a reduction of cholesterol in the blood. Excessive blood pressure (hypertension), underlying many cardiovascular problems, can often be reduced by regular physical exercise.

Smoking and Cardiovascular Diseases

It has been suggested for years that smoking has adverse effects on the cardiovascular system. Studies of large groups of people reinforce this suggestion by showing that cigarette smokers, in particular, are prone to die earlier (in middle age rather than old age) of certain cardiovascular disorders than are nonsmokers. Chief among these disorders is coronary artery disease.

The cardiovascular effects of smoking are those caused by *nicotine* alone. Low concentrations of nicotine (obtained from the smoking of one or two cigarettes) cause in most persons an increase in the resting heart rate of 15 to 25 beats per minute (30,000 extra beats per day), a rise in blood pressure, and an increase in the heart output. As the number of cigarettes smoked increases, there is also constriction in both the coronary arteries and the arteries of the rest of the body. Constriction is easily noted in the fingers after smoking (temperature drops because of a lack of blood). Such decreased blood flow accounts for the association of cigarette smoking and the increased incidence of coronary disease.

If as few as eight cigarettes are smoked within a period of one day, there may be an impairment of the oxygen-carrying mechanism of the blood. Such oxygen reduction in the body reduces the body's ability to produce adequate energy. This affects the total performance of the individual.

Physical Exercise

The term "endurance fitness" describes the ability to engage in prolonged physical activity without undue fatigue or overexertion. Such fitness is some indication of the overall health of the heart and the lungs (in fact, of the entire cardiovascular-respiratory system) — not simply of a person's muscular strength or agility.

It takes two things to create energy for physical activity, food and oxygen. The body stores nutrients, but it cannot store oxygen. During physical activity much of the oxygen of the blood is used up by the contracting muscles. This increases the amount of carbon dioxide (CO_2) in the blood and decreases the available oxygen (O_2). The result of such activity is increased respiration in the lungs, heart rate, and flow of blood throughout the body. During severe exercise, however, the CO_2 concentration accumulates quickly while the body's supply of O_2 dwindles rapidly. After such exertion has stopped, it takes the body some time to get rid of this CO_2 and restore its O_2 supply.

Consequently, a person's fitness may be judged by the efficiency of his oxygen-delivery system, as determined by how few times the heart beats per minute, the size of the openings of the blood vessels, and the pressure of the blood. A well-conditioned heart is able to pump *more* blood with *fewer* beats. (Twenty fewer beats per minute will save a person 30,000 beats per day.) Well-conditioned blood vessels are relatively large and more elastic, creating less resistance and freer routes for blood-oxygen delivery to the body.

The key to physical fitness, therefore, is oxygen consumption. The body needs oxygen to produce energy. Since oxygen cannot be stored, it must be brought in constantly. The more the body can bring in *and* deliver, the better the individual's physical fitness.

Exercise that makes a person "huff and puff" stretches his oxygen-delivery system. By the time he begins to puff, he has reached his maximum rate of oxygen delivery. Regular exercise routines enable us to lengthen the period of time we can exercise before we begin to puff. Exercises that are particularly useful for this are jogging, swimming, cycling, walking, stationary running, and playing handball, basketball, and squash (in this order). Poor exercises include isometrics, weight lifting, and calisthenics (which increase the size of muscles, but do not significantly improve the oxygen-delivery system).

As people age, oxygen delivery becomes less effective and blood pressure rises. Eventually the weakened circulatory system cannot match the work load, and the cardiovascular system breaks down. Then a person is more likely to have a heart attack or stroke and is increasingly vulnerable to many other illnesses.

Other Ways of Preventing Cardiovascular Diseases

The incidence of cardiovascular diseases can be reduced by the following measures:

1. Eat the proper foods in reasonable amounts.
2. Avoid or secure adequate treatment for infection.
3. Avoid excessive emotional upsets.
4. Get adequate and regular rest.
5. Exercise regularly.
6. Have regular periodic physical examinations.

Summary

I. Circulation

   A. Provides continuous and rapid movement of food, water, and oxygen to the cells

   B. Removes wastes from the cells

II. Blood

   A. Obtains oxygen from the lungs, carries foods and wastes to and from cells, and regulates body temperature

B. Components of blood:

    1. Plasma—liquid portion, about 90 percent water

    2. Erythrocytes—red blood cells

    3. Leukocytes—white blood cells

    4. Platelets—fragments of larger cells, important in clotting

C. Blood groups—determined by kind of protein present in red cells

D. Anemias

    1. Conditions in which oxygen-carrying capacity of blood is reduced

    2. Causes include heredity, diet, hemorrhage, or destruction of red blood cells

    3. Sickle cell anemia

        a. Hereditary anemia common among black people

        b. Sickle-shaped red blood cells slow or block circulation through small vessels

        c. Caused by recessive genes

            (1) 1 in 10 black Americans is a carrier

            (2) 1 in 400 black babies has actual disease

        d. Carriers can be detected through blood test

III. The Heart

A. Structure

    1. Double pump with septum dividing right and left sides

    2. Four chambers—left and right atria, left and right ventricles

    3. Three layers—myocardium, endocardium, epicardium

    4. Four valves—tricuspid, pulmonary semilunar, bicuspid (mitral), aortic semilunar

B. Action

    1. Independent beat starts in the sinoatrial node

    2. Impulse next passes to atrioventricular node

    3. Impulse then transmitted to bundle of His

    4. Systole—phase of contraction of ventricles or atria

    5. Diastole—phase of relaxation of ventricles or atria

C. Heartbeat

    1. Rate for person at rest ranges between 70 and 75 beats per minute

    2. Less strenuous for heart to beat fewer times

D. Output:

    1. Adult heart pumps about 5 quarts of blood per minute

    2. Cardiac output does not necessarily relate to rate of heartbeat

E. Blood pressure:

   1. Measured in terms of how high a column of mercury it will replace, first during systole and then during diastole

   2. Should be sufficient to maintain proper circulation, but not excessive so as to burst the arteries

F. Pulse:

   1. Result of pressure on the walls of the arteries

   2. Pulse rate same as heart rate

G. Blood vessels—carry blood throughout the body

   1. Arteries—carry blood away from the heart

   2. Veins—carry blood to the heart

   3. Arterioles—smallest divisions of arteries

   4. Capillaries—smallest vessels of the body; connecting link between arterioles and venules

   5. Venules—smallest divisions of veins

H. Lymphatics:

   1. Intercellular tissue fluid is known as "lymph"

   2. Lymph must be continually drained from tissue space through the lymphatic system.

IV. Types and Causes of Circulatory Diseases

A. Congenital disorders

   1. Maternal illness, X rays, or drugs may cause heart disorders in the unborn child

   2. Lack of oxygenated blood may cause skin to have bluish hue at birth ("blue baby")

   3. Can often be surgically corrected

B. Degenerative cardiovascular disorders —reduction of efficiency of heart

   1. Rheumatic heart disease—antibodies attack endocardium, causing heart valves to become scarred.

   2. Heart murmurs—abnormal sounds produced from improperly working heart valves

   3. Atherosclerosis

      a. Deposit of fatty materials in walls of arteries

      b. Reduces blood flow, leading to:

         (1) Angina pectoris (pains in chest)

         (2) Coronary thrombosis (blood clot in coronary artery)

      (3) Some senility

      (4) Strokes

      (5) Gangrene, especially in feet and legs

      (6) High blood pressure

    c. Possible causes include:

      (1) Excess intake of cholesterol, animal fats, or table sugar

      (2) Emotional stress

      (3) Lack of exercise

  4. Hypertension—high blood pressure

  5. Cerebrovascular accidents—interruption in normal flow of blood to brain (strokes)

  6. Varicose veins—destruction of valves resulting from overstretched veins

  7. Shock—progressive condition caused by reduced blood flow

C. Coronary heart disease:

  1. Blockage of the arteries serving the heart

  2. Pain caused by blood-flow deficiency is called "angina pectoris"

  3. Factors relating to heart disease —heredity, environment, nutrition, and personal health

  4. Symptoms of heart disease—dizziness, chest pain, swelling, breathlessness

  5. Treatment depends on nature of disease and how critical the patient's condition is

    a. Emergency care—person who has just had heart attack must be taken to hospital and possibly given oxygen and drugs

    b. Long-term care—prevent anginal discomfort, help circulation, set up diet, schedule exercise

    c. Bypass surgery—diseased coronary artery bypassed to increase blood supply to heart muscle

V. Prevention of Cardiovascular Diseases

  A. Stop cigarette smoking

  B. Reduce intake of cholesterol

  C. Get regular physical exercise

  D. Eat proper foods in reasonable amounts

  E. Get adequate rest

  F. Avoid emotional upsets

  G. Have periodic physical examinations

Questions for Review

1. What aspects of the American way of life appear to contribute to the high incidence of circulatory disease in the United States today?

2. Name and describe the major components of blood.

3. How can sickle cell anemia be prevented?

4. In a paragraph, trace the circulation of blood from the time it leaves the right atrium until it returns to the right atrium.

5. What is the difference between systolic and diastolic blood pressure? What is the meaning of a blood pressure reading of 120 over 80?

6. Congenital heart disorders often develop during the first three months of fetal life. What are these potential abnormalities and what are their effects?

7. When is an individual most likely to contract rheumatic fever? What kind of damage most commonly occurs as a result of rheumatic fever?

8. What is a heart murmur?

9. Describe the development of atherosclerosis and some of its effects.

10. What is hypertension? What are its effects?

11. What is the difference between a stroke and a heart attack?

12. Studies indicate that there is a direct relationship between smoking and cardiovascular disease. What causes the cardiovascular effects of smoking? What are the effects?

13. What steps can be taken to prevent cardiovascular diseases?

Chapter 6
CANCER

The general term "cancer" includes a group of related diseases that are characterized by the abnormal growth and spread of body cells. Considered as a group, the various types of cancer are the number two cause of death in the United States today. Approximately 1 in every 4 Americans will develop cancer sometime during life. Currently, approximately 18 percent of all deaths in this country are attributed to some form of cancer. This means that about one-third of all cancer patients are now being successfully cured, a fraction that could be raised to one-half merely by application of currently accepted methods of diagnosis and treatment. In actual numbers, over 100,000 additional lives could be saved each year by early diagnosis and prompt treatment of cancer.

Incidence of Cancer

For about 40 years—since 1936—the cancer death rate for women in the United States has slowly declined, with a total drop of about 8 percent. But during the same period the rate for males has increased by about 40 percent. These trends have not been uniform for all types of cancer: Some types are killing more people than 40 years ago while others are killing fewer.

The decline in cancer deaths among women is due mainly to a sharp reduction in deaths from cervical cancer, which can now be readily detected through the "Pap" smear test and successfully treated in its early stages.

The rise in cancer deaths of men is due largely to a *1,400 percent increase* in lung cancer, which is almost entirely a result of increased

TABLE 6.1   Major Cancers in the United States

Type of Cancer	Cases Per Year	Deaths Per Year
Lung	83,000	75,000
Colon and rectum	99,000	48,000
Breast	90,000	33,000
Lymphomas	28,000	20,000
Prostate	54,000	18,000
Kidney and bladder	43,000	16,000
Leukemia	21,000	15,000
Stomach	23,000	14,000
Uterus	46,000	11,000
Mouth and throat	24,000	8,000
Skin	300,000	5,000
Larynx	10,000	3,000

Source: *Cancer Facts and Figures,* 1974 American Cancer Society.

TABLE 6.2   Most Common Fatal Cancers

Age and Sex	Most Common Fatal Cancers
Total, all ages	
Male:	Lung, colon and rectum, prostate, stomach, pancreas
Female:	Breast, colon and rectum, uterus, lung, ovary
Under 15 years	
Male:	Leukemia, brain, lymphosarcoma, bone, kidney
Female:	Leukemia, brain, bone, kidney, lymphosarcoma
15–34 years	Leukemia, Hodgkin's disease, brain, testis,
Male:	lymphosarcoma
Female:	Breast, leukemia, uterus, Hodgkin's disease, brain
35–54	
Male	Lung, colon and rectum, pancreas, brain, stomach
Female:	Breast, uterus, lung, colon and rectum, ovary
55–74	
Male:	Lung, colon and rectum, prostate, pancreas, stomach
Female:	Breast, colon and rectum, lung, uterus, ovary
Over 75 years	
Male:	Prostate, lung, colon and rectum, stomach, pancreas
Female:	Colon and rectum, breast, stomach, pancreas, uterus

Source: Adapted from *Cancer Facts and Figures,* 1974, American Cancer Society.
Note: Listed in decending order of number of actual deaths.

cigarette smoking. Since 1949, more men than women have been dying each year of cancer; the current ratio is about 55 to 45.

The incidence of cancer among blacks is markedly higher than in whites, particularly among men. For unknown reasons, black men show considerably higher rates for cancers of the prostate and esophagus than do white men. Black women have a higher rate of cervical cancer than white women, but lower rates of cancers of the breast and body of the uterus (other than the cervix).

Tables 6.1 and 6.2 summarize the incidence of major cancers and cancer-caused deaths in the United States.

The Nature of Cancer

Throughout a person's life the cells in many parts of the body are constantly dividing to provide replacements for worn-out or damaged cells. In cancer the normal, orderly division and growth of the cells is replaced by rapid, uncontrolled division and growth. In most cases cancer seems to start when a single cell goes wild.

Cancer cells are structurally similar to normal cells; they do show some clear differences, however. The *nucleus* in cancer cells, as well as in normal cells, is where the genetic material (DNA) is found. It is the center of cell reproduction and directs the overall cell functions. Generally, a cancer cell may be distinguished from a normal cell principally by its nucleus. The nucleus of a cancer cell is usually larger than that of a normal cell, and differs in the number and appearance of its chromosomes and in the number of nucleoli present (Figure 6.1). The earliest detectable sign of cancer is an increase in the number of chromosomes in a cell and changes in their shapes.

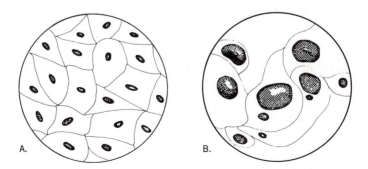

Figure 6.1 *Cancer cells contrasted with normal cells. Cancer cells have larger irregular nuclei and double nuclei, and the cells often take strange shapes. (A) Microscopic view of "Pap" smear to detect cervical cancer showing normal cells. (B) Microscopic view of "Pap" smear to detect cervical cancer showing cancer cells.*

An outstanding characteristic of cancer cells is their *invasive* ability. Normal cells are slowed in dividing by close contact with surrounding cells. But cancer cells do not show such slowing. They continue to divide and push into and invade the surrounding normal tissues.

Another important characteristic of cancer is *metastasis,* the transfer of disease from one organ to another. Cancerous growths tend to shed living cancer cells. These cells can be picked up by the blood or lymph and carried to remote parts of the body. Wherever these cells happen to lodge, they begin to grow, divide, and invade. Thus, through the process of metastasis, the body of the cancer victim may become riddled with dozens of growths at many locations.

Tumors

Any mass of new tissue that persists and grows without serving any useful purpose is called a *tumor* or *neoplasm* (new formation). Tumors are divided into two classes—*benign* (noncancerous) and *malignant* (cancerous). The growth of tumors is characteristic of many, but not all, kinds of cancer.

BENIGN TUMORS

Benign tumors tend to grow more slowly than malignant tumors and are usually surrounded by a fibrous membrane that prevents them from invading surrounding tissues. They do not metastasize (spread into remote parts of the body). They may, however, reach such an enormous size that they exert dangerous pressure on the surrounding organs.

Benign tumors commonly occur on the skin as warts or birthmarks, inside the body as fibrous tumors or cysts, or on the skeleton as growths of bone tissue. Some benign tumors, if exposed to certain harmful irritations (explained later), may become malignant.

MALIGNANT TUMORS

Malignant tumors are cancerous growths. Kinds of cancers may be recognized by their names, which often end in *-oma* (tumor). Some examples: *carcinomas* are malignancies of epithelial tissue; *melanomas* of pigment cells (skin); *lymphomas* of lymph tissue; *sarcomas* of connective tissue; and so forth.

How Cancer Kills

Although cancer can kill in many ways, three conditions most often lead to the death of the cancer victim—*anemia, infection,* and *debility.*

Anemia is the inability of the blood to carry sufficient oxygen in the body. In some types of cancer there is an insufficient production of red blood cells, or red blood cells are produced but do not survive long enough. In other cancers there is internal bleeding that results in a dangerous loss of red blood cells.

Infection often results from the inability of the white blood cells to destroy infectious germs. In some types of cancer few white blood cells are produced. In other cancers, such as leukemia, vast number of white cells are produced, but they are malformed and unable to fight germs.

Debility, the lack or loss of strength, is common in almost all forms of cancer. It may result from simple undernutrition, such as might occur when some part of the digestive system is damaged. Debility may also be a side effect of treatments such as surgery, drugs, or radiation.

Symptoms of Cancer

The degree of success in treating cancer depends largely upon how early the disease is detected and treatment is begun. It is extremely important for everyone to recognize the early symptoms of cancer. They are:

> **1.** *Any sore that does not heal,* regardless of its appearance or location.
> **2.** *Any lump or thickening* anywhere on or in the body.
> **3.** *Any unusual bleeding or discharge* from any body opening.
> **4.** *Any change in a wart, mole, or birthmark,* such as a change in its color or size.
> **5.** *Persistent indigestion or difficulty in swallowing.*
> **6.** *Persistent hoarseness or cough.*
> **7.** *Any change in bowel or urination habits.*
> **8.** *Any unusual pain*—seldom a symptom of early cancer, but not to be ignored.

If any of these symptoms appear, either singly or in combination, a physician should be seen as soon as possible. Any of these symptoms can be produced by many conditions other than cancer, but prompt treatment of cancer is so essential that it is foolish to take a "wait and see" attitude. If cancer is found, it can be promptly treated; if cancer is found not to be present, needless worry can be avoided.

Diagnosis of Cancer

A physician can definitely confirm the presence of cancer in several ways. Some of these methods are applied when a patient notices one of the early symptoms of possible cancer. Others are used on a routine, periodic basis to detect symptomless forms of cancer.

X Rays

Certain cancers, such as lung cancer, may be detected through X rays. It is important that smokers have chest X rays frequently. Some authorities recommend chest X rays every six months for smokers. A special X-ray technique for breast examination is called *mammography.*

Smear Tests

Since many kinds of malignant tumors shed cancer cells from their surface, it is often possible to detect cancer through a microscopic examination of certain body fluids. This is accomplished by smearing the fluid onto a glass microscope slide, staining it, and examining the slide under the microscope.

The most commonly used smear test is the *Papanicolaou* (Pap) *smear test* for cancer of the uterus. In this simple procedure, a microscope slide is prepared by swabbing the cervix. Since most uterine cancer begins on the cervix, which extends into the vagina, cancerous cells may be detected while the uterine cancer is still in its early development.

Uterine cancer usually remains on the cervix for one to two years before it begins its devastating spread through the entire uterus and the surrounding organs. If the cancer is detected through a Pap smear during this early period, the chances of a successful cure are excellent. It is strongly recommended that every woman have a Pap test every year, without fail, starting in her late teens. After age 45, the test should be made every six months.

Blood Tests

Leukemia and other cancers of the blood-forming organs are normally diagnosed through a count of the blood cells on a stained microscope slide. Some progress has been made toward the development of blood tests for other forms of cancer, but it must be emphasized that there is currently no way of detecting many forms of cancer through blood tests.

Rectal Examinations

The lower portion of the large intestine is a common place for cancer to develop. Cancers in this area are usually symptomless in their early stages. But a physician often can detect rectal cancers through a visual inspection of the inner walls of the lower large intestine by means of a special instrument called a *proctoscope* or *sigmoidoscope,* which is inserted through the rectum. This instrument lights the inside of the lower intestine and transmits an image to the physician. Rectal examinations at yearly intervals are highly recommended for all persons over 35 years of age.

Biopsy

A *biopsy* is the microscopic examination of cells removed from a living organ for the purpose of diagnosis. This procedure is normally applied when an organ or tumor is suspected of being cancerous. A small slice of the suspected tissue is removed and examined, often while the patient waits. If the tumor is cancerous, extra care is taken to ensure the complete removal of all accessible cancerous tissue.

Treatment of Cancer

Many people have the mistaken idea that a cancer diagnosis is the same as a death sentence. Actually, with prompt medical treatment the chances of survival are good with many types of cancer. Even when the disease cannot be completely cured, proper treatment often can extend a patient's life.

A true cure of a case of cancer requires that every living cancer cell be killed or removed from the body. Since it cannot be immediately determined whether this has been accomplished, a cancer patient is considered cured only after he has shown no sign of cancer for at least five years after treatment.

There are four principal approaches to the treatment of cancer today—surgery, radiation (the use of X rays or radioactive material), chemotherapy (the use of drugs and hormones), and immunotherapy. Of these methods, surgery and radiation offer the best chances of a cure. A few types of cancer have been cured with drugs, but for most forms of cancer the value of drugs is in prolonging the life of the patient and in relieving associated symptoms, such as pain. Immunotherapy is still largely experimental. A combination of two or more treatment methods may be more effective than any one method alone. In addition, a second or third method is often helpful if the primary treatment fails to cure or halt the growth of cancer.

Surgery

The key to successful treatment of cancer is to diagnose it at a stage when the cancer can be removed entirely from the body. The major use of surgery in the treatment of cancer is to attempt to remove all of the cancerous tissue in the involved area. Because of the spreading nature of cancer, varying amounts of normal tissue are often removed along with the malignant growth. Surgery may be used to remove certain endocrine glands (ovaries, testes, pituitary, or adrenal glands) in an effort to check the spread of cancer in organs that depend on the hormones produced by these glands for growth. It is also used to relieve pain in cases of incurable cancer by severing nerves serving the area of pain.

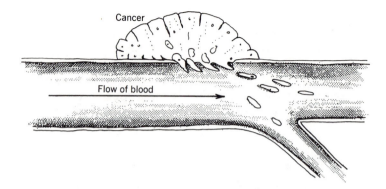

Figure 6.2   *Metastasis (invasion) by cancer into a blood vessel or lymph vessel. Metastasis is the process of transferring cancer from one organ or part of the body to another. The result of such transferring is the formation of new sites (secondary growths) of cancer.*

Surgery, radiation, and chemotherapy are combined in an effort to find the most effective cancer cures possible. Chemicals are now fed directly into surgical wounds to prevent the spread of any remaining cancer cells into the blood or lymph (by metastasis, as shown in Figure 6.2). Preoperative radiation to prevent implantation (Figure 6.3) and growth of tumors in tissue surrounding the surgical area is also used.

Radiation

Radiation has been used as a cancer treatment for about fifty years. Amounts of radiation that seem to have no effect on normal cells cause considerable damage to cancerous cells, and sometimes even destroy the cancer completely. Some types of cancer, however, are not affected by doses of radiation that are safe for normal tissue. Several sources of radiation are used in cancer treatment —*high-voltage x-ray machines* and *radioisotopes* (elements such as cobalt that release energy and nuclear particles as they change to other elements at a predictable rate).

X RAYS

X rays are controlled beams of electrons at variable high-energy levels. X rays of extremely high energy levels readily penetrate tissue and can be used to arrest the growth of or kill cancerous cells in deep internal organs. Low-energy X rays are used for superficial cancers such as skin growths.

RADIOACTIVE COBALT

Radioactive cobalt releases a much more penetrating beam than X rays. Used in a procedure similar to that used with X rays, cobalt

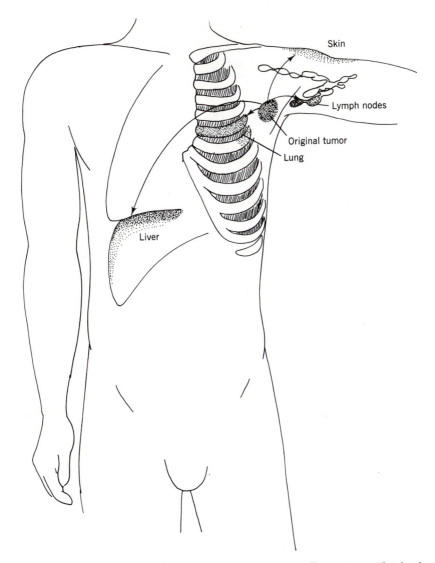

Figure 6.3 *Implantation of cancer. Because cancer cells are so easily shed, they may become dislodged easily and implant themselves in some adjacent organ or area, where they continue to grow and produce their destructive effects.*

therapy involves placing the patient so that he or the cobalt can be rotated during exposure to the radiation beam with the tumor at the center of rotation. This placement and rotation permit a maximum amount of radiation without unnecessary damage to nearby healthy tissue. (A cobalt machine is shown in Figure 6.4.)

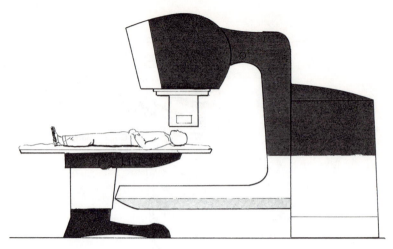

Figure 6.4 *Cobalt machine for radiation therapy.*

RADIOISOTOPES

The advantage of radioisotopes is that they are picked up by the body through the digestive system, like many other chemicals. A physician may select the appropriate radioactive isotope on the basis of the area or organ he wishes to reach. Certain glands and organs tend to collect specific chemicals. As small, harmless doses of a radioisotope are introduced into the body, they accumulate at the area of the tumor. The thyroid gland, for instance, tends to collect and accumulate iodine. Consequently, in the treatment of cancer of the thyroid, a radioisotope of iodine (I^{131}) is introduced into the body and accumulated by the thyroid gland. Its destructive energy is thus concentrated in a strategic spot to attack the tumor.

Chemotherapy

Although surgery or radiation can often remove or arrest localized cancers, rarely can they cure cancers that have spread beyond their point or origin. They cannot be used to cure cancers of the blood or blood-forming tissues which are widespread from the beginning. For many years scientists felt that the only way to treat such cancers would be with drugs or chemicals that would destroy cancer cells and yet not harm normal tissues. Prior to the 1940s, there was no evidence that such drugs could be produced. Today, however, many drugs are being used in the treatment of cancer, and in the past few years progress has been made in the chemotherapy of certain types of cancer, such as leukemia.

These effective drugs, as used by research medical centers and practicing physicians, should not be confused with the unproven cancer remedies that have been marketed for many years. Having failed to gain Food and Drug Administration approval for sale of these remedies in the United States, their promoters have established clinics in Canada, Mexico, and other countries. Many cancer patients travel to these countries to obtain unproven remedies such as Krebiozen. Too often, the time spent trying worthless cancer treatments delays effective treatment until a cure is impossible.

Depending on the type of cancer and its extent, drugs may be used alone or in combination with surgery or radiation. Some drugs attack cancerous cells directly, hormones are important in slowing the growth of certain cancers, and pain relievers are often necessary in advanced cases.

Immunotherapy

One of the newer and more promising approaches to treating cancers is through stimulating the patient's antibody-producing tissues to produce antibodies which attack his cancerous cells. This approach is consistent with the theory that at least some cases of cancer are the result of deficient antibody production. According to this theory cancerous cells periodically appear in everyone. But in most people the immune response is strong enough to destroy tiny cancers as they appear. Dangerous cancers develop only when the antibody production is inadequate to eliminate new cancers as they first arise.

Several means of stimulating antibody production are being tested; none of these is yet considered to be a proven treatment for cancer. One treatment which has shown some promise for certain cancers is the injection of BCG vaccine (for Bacillus Calmette-Guerin, named after the Frenchmen who developed it). BCG is a weakened (attenuated) strain of living tuberculosis bacteria which is routinely used to immunize against tuberculosis in some European countries, but is seldom used in the United States. BCG is not an anticancer drug as such, but it does appear to stimulate the immune system. When injected directly into cancer lesions, it can cause the immune system to send antituberculosis antibodies to the scene to fight the invaders. In some patients, these antibodies apparently attack the cancers as well.

Other experiments have involved vaccines made from tumors similar to those of the patient, injecting the substance into cancer victims in the hope of triggering an immune reaction that is specifically directed against the cancer. Still another immunologic approach has been the transplant of lymphatic (antibody-producing) tissue from healthy persons to cancer patients.

As more and more evidence accumulates linking viruses to at least some forms of cancer, the chance of producing effective specific vaccines against those cancers increases. If specific cancer-causing viruses are isolated, it will probably be only a matter of time until vaccines against them can be produced.

Survival Prospects for Cancer Patients

The survival of cancer patients depends on many factors. One of the most important is the location of the tumor. Other factors include the degree to which the tumor has spread when treatment begins, the age and general health of the patient, and the method of treatment. Figure 6.5 shows how survival during the first five years after diagnosis varies with the site of the tumor. Because of the large number of males who have lung cancer, the survival of males in general is somewhat below the survival rate of females.

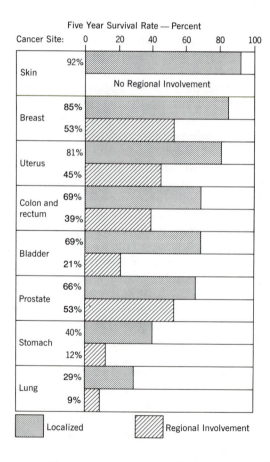

Figure 6.5 *Survival rates for cancer patients during the first five years after diagnosis. From Cancer Facts and Figures, 1974, American Cancer Society.*

Chances for survival are also closely related to the size of the tumor and how much tissue is involved. Patients with strictly localized tumors generally have the best survival rates. The rates usually decrease in direct relation to the advancing tumor stage. However, some people with extremely small and localized cancers die quickly despite apparently adequate treatment, while a very few people with widespread metastasis live for many years with no treatment at all. This phenomenon is unexplained as yet.

Some Important Types of Cancer

Almost any part of the body can become cancerous, but cancer is much more common in some organs than in others. We shall consider several of the more important forms, including those that are important either in number of cases or in number of deaths caused.

Lung Cancer

More people die of lung cancer than of any other type of cancer. The number of victims has risen sharply during the past 30 years, and lung cancer now exceeds automobile accidents as a cause of death, killing about 75,000 persons per year.

The first symptoms of lung cancer—coughing, wheezing, or vague chest pain—are so commonplace that they rarely cause a person to consult a physician or to suspect lung cancer. Thus lung cancer is seldom diagnosed in its early stages.

A chest X ray may reveal lung cancer before any serious symptoms appear. Lung cancer may appear as a shadow that can usually be distinguished by an expert from shadows caused by other lung diseases. When there is doubt about an X ray, microscopic examination of cells found in the sputum may be made on a smear slide, or a biopsy may be taken of the suspected cancerous tissue.

A confirmed case of lung cancer is usually treated by surgery or radiation. The survival rate in lung cancer cases is extremely low, since it is seldom diagnosed early enough to allow the complete surgical removal of all cancerous tissue.

Yet lung cancer is among the most preventable of all cancers. The relationship between it and smoking is clearly and irrefutably established. Although lung cancer is not unknown among nonsmokers, it is many times more common among smokers. It has been statistically established that light smokers have several times as much chance of lung cancer as nonsmokers and that heavy smokers run a much greater risk than light smokers. Cigarette smoking is more likely to result in lung cancer than is cigar or pipe smoking, since an individual is more likely to inhale cigarette smoke than pipe or cigar smoke.

Smoking does not make lung cancer inevitable. Lung cancer is not even the greatest hazard associated with smoking (heart disease is more common). *But the chances of getting lung cancer and many other diseases are greatly increased by heavy smoking.*

The way in which smoking causes lung cancer is fairly well understood today. Tobacco smoke contains hundreds of different chemical compounds that are deposited in the bronchial tubes leading to the lungs and on other tissues in contact with it. At least fifteen of these chemicals are known *carcinogens*—materials that have been proven to cause cancer.

With prolonged exposure to tobacco smoke, the cells of the bronchial tubes gradually change. The surface of the bronchial tubes is normally moist, covered with *mucus* produced by its cells. Many of the surface cells contain small whiplike fringes called *cilia* (see inset, Figure 6.6). These cilia wave back and forth in such a way as to propel the mucus upward and outward toward the throat. Any irritating or poisonous particles entering the bronchial tubes are likely to be trapped in the mucus and propelled by the cilia out of the tubes and into the throat by a cough. This process is a protective mechanism that removes unwanted and irritating materials from the easily damaged lungs.

Cigarette smoke paralyzes this action of the cilia in the bronchial tubes. It causes changes to occur in the lining so that the cilia eventually disappear altogether, depriving the bronchial tubes of this nor-

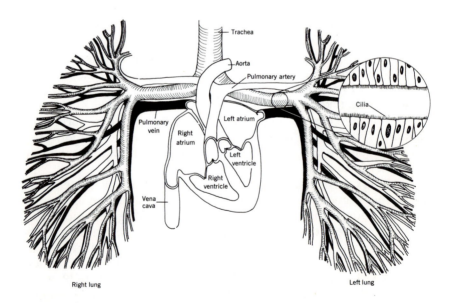

Figure 6.6. *Relative position of heart, lungs, and bronchial tubes. Inset shows cilia lining the bronchial tubes.*

mal protective mechanism. Thus relationships between smoking and lung cancer, as well as many respiratory conditions, are due at least in part to the effects of smoke on the cilia rather than only to the direct action of carcinogens.

Other Tobacco-Related Cancers

In addition to lung cancer, the smoker assumes as increased risk of cancer of the lip, tongue, mouth, throat, and larynx (voice box). These cancers are associated with all forms of tobacco usage, including cigarettes, pipes, cigars, and chewing tobacco. The risk of lip, tongue, and mouth cancers is greater with pipes and cigars than with cigarettes.

The symptoms of these forms of cancer include a sore that does not heal, swallowing difficulty, and hoarseness. With prompt treatment, the chance of successfully curing any of these cancers is good.

Breast Cancer

Breast cancer is the leading cause of cancer death among women. Among women in the age group of 15 to 74, it is the most common single cause of death. About 90,000 cases are discovered each year in the United States, and almost 33,000 women die yearly of breast cancer. Nearly 4 percent of all women eventually develop breast cancer.

Although there is no known way of preventing breast cancer, it need not result in death if diagnosed and treated promptly. It has been estimated that the survival rate (now over 50 percent) could be increased considerably if every woman were more alert to the early symptoms of breast cancer. These symptoms include any abnormal lump or thickening in the breast or any unusual discharge from the nipple.

Every woman should examine her breasts for cancer symptoms monthly, immediately following her menstrual period. Examination during the menstrual period is unsatisfactory because of the temporary changes and tenderness that normally may occur in the breasts at this time. The procedure of breast self-examination is outlined in Figure 6.7. Further information may be obtained from a physician or from the American Cancer Society. Also, as shown in Figure 6.8, mammography (a special type of X-ray examination of the breast for tumors too small to be felt) is used very successfully in the diagnosis of breast cancer.

Cancer of the Uterus

Cancer of the uterus is the second most common cause of cancer death among women. Deaths from uterine cancer have decreased over 50 percent in the last 25 years as a result of early detection of

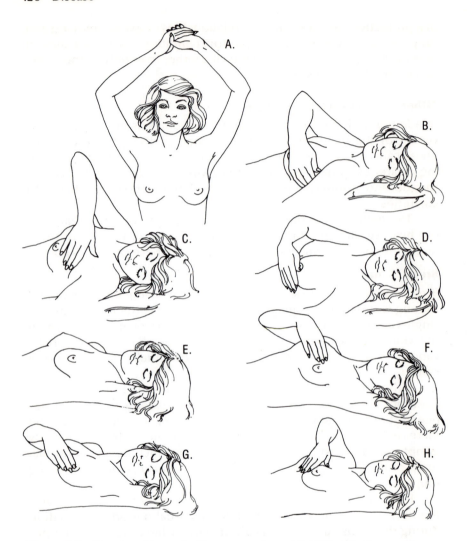

Figure 6.7 *Breast self-examination procedure. (A) Sitting before a mirror, arms at the sides and posture erect, the breasts are examined for symmetry in size and shape, noting any dimpling of the skin or retraction of the nipple. With arms over head, these observations are repeated. (B) With padding in place under the shoulder and arm at the side, the woman begins by carefully feeling the tissues that extend well into the armpit area. Any lump or thickening is noted. (C) The woman now proceeds to inspect the upper, outer portion of the breast. She makes use of the sensitive flats of her fingers instead of their tips, and she gives this portion special attention. Again, any lump or thickening is noted. (D) Having covered the armpit region and the upper, outer portion, the woman now goes over the remainder of the outer half of the breast, feeling in successive stages from the outer margin to the*

nipple. Lumps or thickenings are noted. (E) When the entire outer half of the breast has been examined, with the arm at her side, the woman now raises the arm over her head. This spreads and thins the tissue for the remaining steps. (F) Beginning at the breastbone, she gently presses the tissue of the inner half of the breast against the chest wall, moving in a series of steps from the breastbone to the middle of the breast. (G) At this point, the woman carefully palpates the nipple area and the tissues lying beneath it. Using the flats of her fingers still, she notes the normal structures of her breast, and any new lumps. (H) She now completes her examination of this breast by feeling the rest of the inner half systematically. Along the lower margin she will find a ridge of firm tissue, which is normal and should not alarm her. Any new lumps or thickenings which she had not noted in the past should be reported to her physician. (National Cancer Institute, Public Health Service, Department of Health, Education and Welfare.)

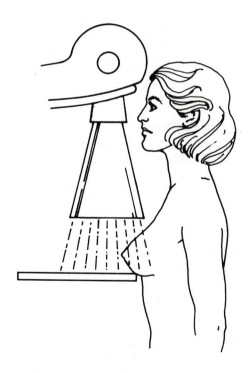

Figure 6.8 *Mammography, a type of X-ray examination of the breast for the presence of tumors too small to be felt. Mammograms of each breast are taken from several angles.*

many cases through Pap smear tests. If more women were to have annual Pap tests, the death rate could be reduced sharply from the current level of about 11,000 per year.

There are no early symptoms of uterine cancer. It usually starts on the cervix of the uterus and tends to remain localized for some time before spreading into other tissues. Therefore a woman who has a Pap smear test every year is likely to discover any possible uterine cancer while it is still localized and can be easily removed. For this reason, every woman, from the late teens on, should have a Pap smear test every year without fail.

Many cancer authorities now believe that cervical cancer is caused by a sexually transmitted virus—herpes simplex, type 2. Several factors support this idea. First, the virus is usually present in cancerous cells from the cervix, though this does not prove any cause-and-effect relationship. Second, women having cervical cancer are more likely to carry type 2 herpes virus than women without cervical cancer, though many cancer free women do carry the virus. Finally, there are several statistical associations between cervical cancer and a woman's sexual history. Virgin women have a very low incidence of cervical cancer; the incidence is higher among women who became sexually active at younger ages; and the incidence increases in relation to the number of different sexual partners. These facts suggest, but do not prove, that cervical cancer results from a sexually transmitted virus.

Cancer of the Colon and Rectum
Cancers of the colon and rectum (lower large intestine) rank high as causes of cancer death among both sexes. Like many other cancers, these occur most often in older persons, but are also an occasional problem in younger people as well. In total number of annual deaths, cancers of the lower large intestine are second only to lung cancer.

The symptoms of these cancers often include rectal bleeding or a change in bowel movement habits. Cancer of the lower large intestine can frequently be detected while in a curable stage when rectal examination procedures are included in routine annual medical checkups. (See page 118.)

Stomach Cancer
For some unknown reason, the incidence of stomach cancer fortunately has dropped 50 percent in the past 20 years. The rate of successful cures for stomach cancer is low, however, because it is seldom detected in its early stages. The first symptom of stomach cancer is usually persistent indigestion, but the cancer has often reached other organs before this symptom is noticed. No prevention is known for cancers of the stomach or lower large intestine.

Prostate Cancer

The *prostate* is one of the fluid-producing glands in the male reproductive system. It is located just below the urinary bladder, and the
tube (urethra) that carries urine from the bladder passes through it.
Cancer of the prostate accounts for about 9 percent of male cancer
deaths. Most of the men affected are elderly.

The cure rate for prostate cancer is low because it is seldom
diagnosed early enough for complete removal of all cancerous tissue.
The first symptom is usually difficulty in urination, a condition common among elderly men because of noncancerous enlargement of
the prostate. Since this symptom is so common, it seldom leads to an
early diagnosis. No prevention for prostate cancer is known.

Skin Cancer

Skin cancer is the most common cancer, but since the rate of successful cures is high, it accounts for relatively few deaths. This high cure
rate can be explained by the fact that skin cancer occurs on the
surface of the body where it is readily visible while still in its early
stages.

A skin cancer may resemble an open sore that does not heal, or it
may look like a wart, mole, or birthmark that has changed its color or
begun to increase in size. If skin cancer is treated as soon as it
appears, the chances of a complete cure are excellent.

The most common cause of skin cancer is excessive exposure to
the sun. Common sites for skin cancer include the face, ears, neck,
arms, and hands, although it may occur anywhere on the body. Skin
cancer is unusually common among persons whose occupations give
them much exposure to the sun. Such occupations include farming,
surveying, fishing, and certain construction trades.

Skin cancer is more prevalent in fair-skinned individuals than in
those with more natural pigmentation. It is especially prevalent
among those whose skin does not tan but burns easily and repeatedly
when exposed to the sun.

Much skin cancer can be prevented by avoiding excess exposure
to the sun. This is especially important for those with more susceptible skin types. Death from skin cancer can be prevented by prompt
medical examination of any suspicious skin condition and prompt
removal of any growths proven to be cancerous.

Leukemia

Leukemia is a cancer of the blood-forming tissues. It is characterized
by the release into the bloodstream of vast numbers of immature
white blood cells. Among all the various types of cancers, leukemia is
the most prevalent among young persons, although it occurs among
all age groups. In persons under 25 years years of age it usually takes

the form of *acute* leukemia, which, untreated, may lead to death in a short time. In persons over 25, leukemia more often occurs in a *chronic* form which may allow survival for many years.

Many persons with leukemia experience periods of *remission* during which the symptoms of the disease partially or even completely disappear. These remissions may be spontaneous or the result of treatments received. After several months or years, however, the symptoms usually reappear.

Much progress has been made in treating leukemia. New drugs and combinations of drugs are constantly being tested. Some drug combinations have prolonged the life of leukemia patients for more than 10 years. In some medical centers, remissions are being achieved in up to 90 percent of childhood leukemia cases. In 1960, only a few patients could be expected to live for five years following the onset of leukemia. Today, about 25 percent of treated patients live that long, and new drugs are constantly extending the life expectancy of leukemia patients.

Causes of Cancer

Before cancer can be conquered, science must gain an understanding of its underlying causes. In recent years, much progress has been made toward this understanding, and intensive research continues to yield new knowledge.

Cancer "Triggers"

Several forces are known to produce cancer with prolonged exposure to human tissues. These forces are often referred to as causes of cancer, but until their role in producing cancer is clarified, it seems preferable to refer to them as "triggers" of cancer. It is quite possible that they only serve to activate some more basic cause. In general, these triggers require prolonged or repeated tissue exposure for cancer to result.

CHEMICAL CARCINOGENS

Hundreds of chemicals have been definitely proved to be *carcinogenic* (cancer causing), either to man or to experimental animals. Some of these carcinogens are contained in tobacco smoke and the smoke from other burning vegetation. Others are carried by various petroleum derivatives such as tars, asphalts, and oils; coal derivatives; and soot.

SUNLIGHT

The factor in sunlight that causes skin cancer is its ultraviolet radiation. Since ultraviolet has little penetrating power, it is not associated with cancers of the deeper tissues.

EXTERNAL IRRITATION

Some cases of cancer seem to be the result of prolonged irritation, such as the constant rubbing of a tight belt or brassiere strap over a wart, mole, or birthmark or the constant rubbing of loose dentures and bridges against the jaw.

EXTREME HEAT

Prolonged exposure to hot objects seems to be an occasional cause of cancer. The high temperature of a pipe stem may be one factor contributing to lip cancer, which so often develops in pipe smokers.

RADIATION

It has been well established that exposure to excessive X rays and other forms of radiation increases the chances of cancer. It has been found that either a single exposure to a high level of radiation or repeated exposure to more moderate levels increases the risk of leukemia. It must be stressed that medical and dental X rays present very little risk. The risk involved in these X rays (which may be used to detect tuberculosis, fractured bones, dangerously infected teeth, and so on) is far less than the risk in not taking them.

Basic Causes of Cancer

Research today is mainly directed toward uncovering the more basic causes of cancer. *How* do the various triggers cause cancer? What about the many cases with no apparent trigger?

HEREDITY

Only a few uncommon forms of cancer are definitely hereditary. One type of cancer of the eye follows a definite hereditary pattern. Several other forms of cancer, while not definitely hereditary, do seem to be unusually common in certain family lines, suggesting that the tendency toward these cancers may be inherited. Examples of these cancers include colon cancer and breast cancer.

MUTATIONS

A *mutation* is a change in the genetic makeup of a cell. When a cell becomes cancerous, definite changes occur in its nucleus and chromosomes (genetic carriers). It is possible that the effect of carcinogenic chemicals and radiation is to alter the hereditary material (DNA). Both radiation and chemicals are known to produce mutations. Some cancers could even be caused by spontaneous mutations, which normally occur in about one of every one million cells.

VIRUSES

A growing mass of evidence suggests that viruses are related to some types of human cancers. There is strong presumptive evidence (though no definite proof) that viruses are involved in leukemia and cervical (uterine) cancer. The exact role of viruses in causing cancer is still unknown.

The association of viruses to cancers raises the question of the communicable nature of cancer—can it ever be "caught"? There is currently no evidence of communicability for the great majority of types of cancer. The one cancer for which there is some presumptive evidence of communicability is cervical cancer. As previously discussed, some authorities now believe that cervical cancer is the result of a sexually transmitted herpes simplex virus.

DEFICIENCIES IN THE IMMUNE MECHANISM

As mentioned in the discussion of cancer treatment, some experts now believe that some forms of cancer are the result of a deficiency in the antibody-producing mechanism. According to this theory, which is supported by some experimental evidence, tiny cancers start from time to time in all of us. But in most people these cancerous cells are destroyed by antibodies before they can develop into life-threatening malignancies. Dangerous cancers develop only when antibody production is inadequate.

None of these possible causes of cancer are mutually exclusive. It is possible that several or even all of them act at one time or another, that different kinds of cancers have different basic causes, and that several factors might contribute to the development of a single type of cancer, perhaps even working together to produce a particular case of cancer in one individual. For example, it is entirely possible that some type of cancer is caused by a virus which most or even all people carry, but which can lead to cancer only in people with deficient antibody production.

In any case, our knowledge of the basic causes of cancer is now expanding at such a rapid rate that it is possible to become optimistic over the possibilities of major breakthrough discoveries on the prevention and treatment of cancer within the next few years.

Summary

I. Incidence of Cancer

    A. Second greatest cause of death in the United States.

    B. Cancer death rate is decreasing in women, increasing in men.

    C. Most important increase is in lung cancer.

    D. Incidence is higher among blacks than among whites

II. The Nature of Cancer

    A. Abnormal growth and spread of body cells

B. Structure of cancer cells

    1. Nucleus of cancer cell usually larger than that of a normal cell

    2. Chromosomes in cancer cell are of abnormal number and shape.

    3. Outstanding characteristic of cancer cells is their invasive ability.

    4. Another characteristic is metastasis—transfer of disease from one organ to another.

C. Tumors—any mass of new tissue that persists and grows wtihout serving any useful purpose.

    1. Benign tumors—do not metastasize

    2. Malignant tumors—cancerous growths

        a. Carcinomas—malignancies of epithelial tissue

        b. Melanomas—malignancies of pigment cells (skin)

        c. Lymphomas—malignancies of lymph tissue

        d. Sarcomas—malignancies of connective tissue

D. Cancer kills by:

    1. Anemia

        a. Insufficient production of red blood cells

        b. Production of red blood cells that do not survive long

        c. Internal bleeding that results in loss of red blood cells

    2. Infection

        1. Insufficient production of white blood cells

        2. White blood cells are malformed and unable to fight germs

    3. Debility

        1. Damage to part of the digestive system

        2. Side effect of surgery, drugs, or radiation

III. Symptoms of Cancer

    A. Any sore that does not heal

    B. Any lump or thickening

    C. Any unusual bleeding or discharge

    D. Any change in wart, mole, or birthmark

    E. Persistent indigestion or difficulty in swallowing

    F. Persistent hoarseness or cough

    G. Any change in bowel or urination habits

    H. Any unusual pain

IV. Diagnosis of Cancer

    A. X rays

    B. Smear tests

    C. Blood tests

    D. Rectal examinations

    E. Biopsy—microscopic examination of cells removed from living organ for purpose of diagnosis

V. Treatment of Cancer

    A. Prompt treatment greatly increases chance of survival.

    B. Surgery

        1. To remove all cancerous tissue

        2. To remove glands in an effort to check the spread of cancer in organs that depend on the hormones produced by these glands

        3. To relieve pain in incurable cases by severing specific nerves

    C. Radiation

        1. X rays

        2. Radioactive cobalt

        3. Radioisotopes

    D. Chemotherapy—many drugs are used today

    E. Immunotherapy

        1. Researchers are trying various methods of stimulating production of anticancer antibodies.

        2. May eventually have vaccines against cancers

VI. Survival Prospects for Cancer Patients

    A. Most important factor is location of tumor

    B. Size of tumor and amount of tissue involved also important

VII. Some Important Types of Cancer

    A. Lung cancer—relationship to smoking has been clearly and irrefutably established.

        1. Symptoms—cough, wheeze, chest pain

        2. Diagnosis—chest X rays, examination of cells in sputum, biopsy

        3. Treatment—surgery or radiation

    B. Other tobacco-related cancers—lip, tongue, mouth, throat, and larynx

        1. Symptoms—sore that does not heal, swallowing difficulty, hoarseness

        2. With prompt treatment, chances of cure are good

C. Breast cancer

    1. Leading cause of cancer death among women

    2. Early detection greatly increases survival rate

    3. Symptoms—abnormal lump or thickening of breast or unusual discharge from nipple

D. Cancer of the uterus:

    1. Usually starts on cervix

    2. Detectable in early stages by Pap smear test

    3. No early symptoms

    4. Possibly caused by sexually transmitted virus

E. Cancer of the colon and rectum

    1. Symptoms—change in bowel habits or rectal bleeding

    2. Rectal examinations included in annual medical checkups help early detection

F. Stomach cancer

    1. First symptom usually persistent indigestion

    2. No prevention known

    3. Incidence has decreased sharply

G. Prostate cancer

    1. First symptom usually difficulty in urination

    2. No prevention known

H. Skin cancer—commonly caused by excessive exposure to sun

    1. May resemble an open sore or a wart, mole, or birthmark that changes color or size

    2. With prompt treatment, chances for cure are excellent

I. Leukemia—cancer of blood-forming tissues

    1. Present throughout body

    2. Treatment includes radiation and specific drugs that act against white blood cells and the blood-forming organs that produce these cells

VIII. Causes of Cancer

  A. "Triggers"

    1. Chemical carcinogens

    2. Sunlight—ultraviolet radiation

    3. External irritation

    4. Extreme heat—such as very high temperature of pipe stem

    5. Radiation

B. Cancer research is focusing on more basic causes of cancer, questioning such factors as:

   1. Heredity

   2. Mutations

   3. Viruses

   4. Deficiencies in the immune mechanism

Questions for Review

   1. What does the term "cancer" mean? What proportion of the people in the United States develop some form of cancer? Do all of them die from it?

   2. Tumors are divided into what two classes? In what ways are they alike? Different?

   3. Define "anemia," "infection," and "debility." What do they have in common as they relate to cancer?

   4. The symptoms of cancer have been widely publicized because of the importance to everyone of their early recognition. What are these early symptoms? Why is early treatment essential?

   5. What methods are available for the detection and diagnosis of cancer? How does a doctor decide which method to use?

   6. A wide variety of treatments and cures for cancer have been tried for many years, but only four are in use today. What are they and how are they used?

   7. What are the prospects of survival for cancer patients? What factors relate to the chances for survival?

   8. Which type of cancer is the most common cause of death? Which is the most preventable?

   9. What is the name given to the chemicals in tobacco smoke that are known to cause lung cancer? What changes take place in the body as a result of smoking? What other kinds of cancer are associated with tobacco use?

10. How can the early symptoms of cancer of the breast, uterus, colon, and rectum be detected?

11. Which is the most prevalent of all cancers? Why is the cure rate for this cancer so high?

12. Which is the most prevalent type of cancer among young persons? How is it treated?

13. What are the "triggers" of cancer? What are the possible basic causes of cancer that researchers are now investigating?

GLOSSARY

active immunity A form of acquired immunity to a disease that results from a person's production of antibodies in response to the presence in his body of antigens, either in the pathogen (germ) or in a vaccine.

acute Having a sudden onset and a short duration.

agglutination The clumping together of blood cells, bacteria, or other small structures.

alveoli Microscopic air sacs within the lungs.

anaphylactic shock A massive allergic reaction including often-fatal circulatory and respiratory failure.

anemia A condition in which there is a decrease in the oxygen-carrying capacity of the blood.

aneurysm A saclike bulging of the wall of an artery or vein that results from weakening of the wall by disease or abnormal development.

angina pectoris Pains in the chest, and often in the left arm and shoulder, caused by insufficient blood supply to the heart muscle.

antibiotic A chemical produced by a microorganism and capable of inhibiting the growth of other microorganisms.

antibody	A protein formed by the lymphatic tissue of the body to destroy or inactivate a specific antigen.
antigen	A foreign substance, usually a protein, which stimulates the production of antibodies.
antitoxin	An antibody that neutralizes the toxin of a bacterium.
aorta	The main artery, which carries blood from the left ventricle of the heart to all parts of the body except the lungs.
arterioles	The smallest arterial vessels after repeated branching of the arteries.
artery	Any one of a system of tubes or vessels which carry blood from the heart.
arthritis	Inflammation of a joint.
arthropod	An insect or insectlike animal.
asthma	A disease in which there are periodic attacks of difficulty in breathing because of a narrowing of the bronchioles.
atherosclerosis	The deposition or formation of yellowish plaques of cholesterol within the arteries.
atrioventricular node (AV node)	A small mass of special muscular fibers, located in the septum between the right atrium and ventricle, which forms the beginning of the bundle of His. It receives an electrical impulse from the sinoatrial node.
atrium	One of the two upper chambers of the heart.
attenuation	The act of weakening, such as the weakening of a pathogen or toxin.
bacillus (pl. bacilli)	A rod-shaped bacterium.
bacteria	Microscopic, single-celled, plantlike organisms.
BCG vaccine	A preparation of living attenuated tuberculosis bacteria used to produce active immunity against tuberculosis (Bacillus Calmette-Guerin).

benign	Not cancerous; not malignant.
bicuspid valve	A valve located between the upper and lower chambers in the left side of the heart; also called "mitral valve."
biopsy	The microscopic examination of cells removed from a living organ for the purpose of diagnosis.
blood	The fluid that circulates through the heart, arteries, capillaries, and veins, carrying nutrients and oxygen to the body cells.
blood type	The classification of red blood cells according to certain proteins they possess.
booster	A dose of vaccine or toxoid administered some time after the original immunization in order to maintain immunity.
bronchioles	Small tubes that carry air into the microscopic air sacs in the lungs.
bronchitis	Inflammation of the bronchioles.
bundle of His	A bundle of specialized muscular fibers that runs from the AV node along the septum down to the lower heart chambers; serves to conduct electrical impulses to the ventricles.
cancer	An abnormal growth and invasive spread of body cells, often characterized by the formation of secondary growths.
capillary	One of the very small tubes or vessels forming a network between the arterioles and the venules. Materials leave and enter the blood through the walls of capillaries.
carcinogen	A substance that causes cancer.
carcinoma	Cancer arising from an epithelial tissue, such as the skin or mucous membrane.
cardiovascular diseases	Diseases affecting the heart and blood vessels.
cerebrovascular accidents	Abnormalities occurring in the arteries of the brain; strokes.

cervix   The necklike lower end of the uterus.

chancre   The primary lesion of syphilis, developing at the exact spot where infection took place.

chemotherapy   The use of drugs or chemicals to treat disease.

cholesterol   A fatty substance found in animal tissue. An excess amount in the blood is often associated with high risk of coronary atherosclerosis.

chromosome   A small rod-shaped structure found in the nucleus of a cell, which contains the genetic material of the cell.

chronic   Occurring over a long period of time.

cilia   Microscopic hairlike structures attached to the surface of cells.

circulation   Movement of blood through the heart and blood vessels of the body.

coccus (pl. cocci) A spherical bacterium.

coma   A state of unconsciousness from which a person cannot be aroused, even by powerful stimulation.

communicable diseases   Diseases that are capable of being transmitted from one person to another.

congenital   Pertaining to presence at birth, resulting from heredity or prenatal environment.

congenital immunity A form of passive immunity which is present in the newborn infant as a result of antibodies that cross the placenta from the blood of the mother into the blood of the fetus.

conjunctivitis   Inflammation of the conjunctiva, the membrane lining the inner surface of the eyelid and the front part of the eyeball.

contagious   Capable of being transmitted directly from one person to another.

convalescence   Period of recovery from a disease.

coronary circulation Circulation of the blood through the blood vessels on the surface of the heart.

coronary occlusion	The closing, or clogging, of the coronary blood vessels of the heart.
debility	Lack or loss of strength.
diabetes	The condition characterized by a deficiency of the hormone insulin.
diabetic coma	A potentially fatal loss of consciousness caused by acidity of the body fluids as a result of inadequately treated diabetes.
diastole	The period of dilation of the heart in each heartbeat.
DPT vaccine	A vaccine containing a mixture of diphtheria, whooping cough, and tetanus vaccines.
embolus	A blood clot (or other substance such as air, fat, tumor) inside a blood vessel which is carried in the bloodstream to a smaller vessel where it becomes an obstruction to circulation.
emphysema	Loss of elasticity and tearing of the minute air sacs of the lungs.
endocarditis	Inflammation of the endocardium usually associated with acute rheumatic fever or some infectious agent.
endocardium	The inner layer of the heart wall.
enzyme	A substance, secreted by living cells, which has the ability to produce chemical changes in some specific substance.
erythrocyte	A red blood cell.
fibrinogen	A soluble protein in the blood which, by the action of certain enzymes, is converted into the insoluble protein of a blood clot.
fibrin threads	Insoluble threads formed in the clotting of blood.
fungus	A filamentous plant which never contains chlorophyll.
gamma globulins	Proteins that are found in the plasma and may be used for the prevention or treatment of certain diseases. Most antibodies are gamma globulins.

general adaptation syndrome	A group of physical reactions elicited by any stressor.
gonococcus (pl. gonococci)	The spherical bacterium which causes gonorrhea.
gout	The deposit of urate crystals in and around the joints.
heart-lung machine	An instrument used to take over the functions of the heart and lungs during corrective surgery on the heart.
hemoglobin	The oxygen-carrying red pigment of the red blood corpuscles.
hemorrhage	A copious discharge of blood from a blood vessel.
hepatitis	Inflammation of the liver.
herpes simplex viruses	A group of viruses causing a variety of lesions ranging from fever blisters, possibly, to certain cancers.
hormone	A chemical substance produced by one of the glands of the body for use elsewhere within the body.
hypertension	Abnormally high blood pressure.
immunity	The ability a person may acquire to resist an infection as a result of producing specific antibodies.
immunization	The process of rendering a person immune.
immunotherapy	Treatment or prevention of disease by means of antigens or antigenic preparations.
incidence	Rate of occurrence.
incubation period	The interval between infection and the appearance of the first symptoms of a disease.
infection	Invasion of the body by pathogens.
infectious	Capable of being communicated by infection; capable of being transmitted.
inferior vena cava	The large vein which empties blood from the legs,

pelvis, and abdomen into the right atrium of the heart.

insulin	A hormone produced by the pancreas and secreted into the blood, where it aids the movement of glucose through cell membranes.
insulin shock	Progressive trembling, convulsions, and coma resulting from an overdose of insulin.
interferon	A chemical released from virus-infected cells to protect other cells from virus infection.
jaundice	A yellowing of the skin due to the deposit of bile pigment, often indicating impaired liver function.
Koplik's spots	Small, irregular bluish-white spots surrounded by red circular areas which are found on the tongue and mouth lining, and are indicative of early measles.
latent	Concealed; hidden; dormant.
lesion	Any pathological or traumatic (injurious) break in tissue.
leukemia	An often fatal disease of the blood-forming organs characterized by a marked increase in the number of leukocytes in the blood.
leukocyte	A white blood cell.
leukocytosis	An increase in the number of leukocytes in the blood.
leukopenia	A reduction in the number of leukocytes in the blood.
lumen	The interior channel of any tubelike organ.
lymph	Tissue fluid confined to vessels and nodes of the lymphatic system.
lymph nodes	Small oval collections of lymphatic tissue interposed in the course of lymphatic vessels.
lymphocytes	A form of small white blood cells.
lymphoma	A general term applied to any type of cancer of the lymphoid tissue.

lysozyme	A substance in tears which inhibits bacteria.
malignant	Cancerous; having the ability to invade; tending to become progressively worse.
mammography	X-ray examination of the breasts.
melanoma	A tumor made of darkly pigmented cells.
metabolic antagonist	A substance that interferes with the chemical processes of life.
metastasis	The transfer of disease from one organ to another.
microbe	A microscopic organism.
microorganism	A microscopic organism; microbe.
monocyte	A large type of white blood cell.
murmur	The sound produced by the backflow of blood through a leaking heart valve.
mutation	A change in the genetic makeup of a cell.
myocardium	The muscular wall of the heart. The heart muscle.
neoplasm	Any new and abnormal growth such as a tumor.
noncommunicable disease	Disease that cannot be transmitted from one person to another.
nucleus	An oval structure within a cell which controls the cell's activities.
occlusion	The closing or blocking of a passage, such as a blood vessel.
organism	A living thing.
osteoarthritis	Degeneration of a joint.
Papanicolaou (Pap) test	The microscopic examination of a specially stained slide prepared for the detection of cancer of the cervix of the uterus.
parasite	A plant or animal that lives on or in another organism (the host) at the expense of the host.

paresis	Partial or incomplete paralysis.
passive immunity	A temporary form of acquired immunity which results from the introduction of antibodies into the blood after their production in some other person or animal.
pathogen	A disease-producing organism or substance.
pericardium	The sac that surrounds the heart.
peritonitis	Inflammation of the peritoneum, the membrane lining the abdominal cavity.
pertussis	Whooping cough.
phagocytosis	The process whereby certain white blood cells and other phagocytic body cells engulf bacteria, dead cells, and other foreign matter.
plasma	The cell-free fluid portion of uncoagulated blood.
platelets	Roundish discs, smaller than red blood cells, found in the blood and associated with clotting.
proctoscope	An instrument for examination of the rectum.
prodromal period	The period of appearance of nonspecific symptoms indicating the approach of a disease.
prostate	A gland in the male, located just beneath the urinary bladder, contributing seminal fluid.
prothrombin	A protein present in plasma and necessary for blood coagulation.
protozoa	Single-celled (usually microscopic) animals.
pulmonary artery	The large artery which conveys unoxygenated (venous) blood from the right ventricle of the heart to the lungs.
pulmonary circulation	Circulation of the blood through the lungs, the flow being from the right ventricle of the heart, through the lungs, back to the left atrium of the heart.
pulse	The expansion and contraction of an artery; may be felt with the finger.

radioisotopes	Elements with radioactive properties.
relapse	The return of the symptoms of a disease after an apparent recovery.
remission	A temporary abatement of the symptoms of a disease.
reservoir	A source of pathogens such as a symptomless carrier or an animal.
rheumatoid arthritis	Inflammation and swelling of the joint.
rubella	German or "three-day" measles.
rubeola	Measles.
sarcoma	Cancer arising from a connective tissue such as bone, cartilage, or lymphatic tissue.
sclerosis	A hardening of body tissues, usually as the result of an accumulation of fibrous tissue.
semilunar valves	Cup-shaped valves.
senility	The physical and mental infirmity of old age.
septum	A dividing wall.
serum	1. The clear liquid which separates from a clot in coagulation. 2. Blood serum from animals that have been inoculated with bacteria or their toxins.
sigmoidoscope	An instrument for the examination of the lower large intestine.
sinoatrial node (SA node)	A small mass of specialized cells that is located in the right upper chamber of the heart and gives rise to the electrical impulses that initiate contractions of the heart. Also called the "pacemaker."
sphygmomanometer	An instrument used for measuring blood pressure within the arteries.
spirillum (pl. spirilla)	A spiral-shaped bacterium; spirochete.
spirochete	A spiral-shaped bacterium.

stenosis	A narrowing or stricture of an opening.
stethoscope	An instrument used to listen to heart and other chest sounds.
stress	A group of changes within a person resulting from the imposition on the person of any harmful external force, or stressor.
stressor	Any force which produces stress.
stroke	An impeded blood supply to part of the brain caused by a clot, hemorrhage, embolus, or other disorder; a cerebrovascular accident.
superior vena cava	The large vein which empties blood from the head, neck, upper arms, and chest into the right atrium of the heart.
symptom	Evidence of some disease or condition.
syndrome	A group of symptoms.
systemic	Affecting the whole body.
systemic circulation	Circulation of the blood through all parts of the body except the lungs, the flow being from the left ventricle of the heart, through the body, back to the right atrium of the heart.
systole	The period of contraction of the heart in each heart beat.
tetanus	1. Continuous steady contraction of a muscle. 2. An infectious disease caused by the toxin of *Clostridium tetani,* resulting in tetanus in various body muscles.
thrombocyte	A blood platelet.
thromboplastin	A substance formed during and essential to the process of blood clotting.
thrombus	A blood clot that forms inside a blood vessel or the cavity of the heart.
toxin	A poison.

toxoid
A weakened bacterial toxin that has lost its toxic properties while retaining its ability to cause the production of antibodies; used in immunization.

transmission
The transfer of something, as of a disease.

tricuspid valve
A valve located between the upper and lower chambers in the right side of the heart.

trivalent vaccine
A vaccine containing three types of antigens.

tubercle
A small rounded nodule produced in tuberculosis infections.

tuberculin
A sterile liquid extracted from the tuberculosis bacterium for use in skin testing for tuberculosis.

tumor
A mass of new tissue which persists and grows without serving any useful purpose.

urethra
The duct carrying urine from the urinary bladder to the exterior of the body.

varicose vein
A permanent enlargement, or distention, of a vein. Often observed as dark markings beneath the skin of the legs.

vector
An animal, usually an arthropod, which transmits pathogens from one host to another.

vein
Any of a series of vessels of the vascular system which carries blood from the various parts of the body back to the heart.

venereal
Related to or transmitted by sexual intercourse.

ventricle
One of the two lower chambers of the heart.

venule
A very small vein.

vessel
A tube circulating a body fluid, as a blood vessel or a lymph vessel.

virus
A minute infectious particle consisting of a core of genetic material (DNA or RNA) contained within a protein coat. All viruses are intracellular parasites.

BIBLIOGRAPHY

American Heart Association, 44 E. 23rd St., New York, Various Publications: *Heart Attack, Heart Disease Caused by Coronary Atherosclerosis, The Framingham Heart Study, Heart Disease in Children, High Blood Pressure, Heart Diseases and Pregnancy, Varicose Veins.*

Andersen, Linda E., "Sickle Cell Anemia," *California's Health*, Vol. 29, No. 5, November 1971.

Benenson, Abram S. (ed.), *Control of Communicable Diseases in Man*, New York, The American Public Health Association, 1970.

Brock, Thomas D., *Biology of Microorganisms*, 2nd ed., Englewood Cliffs, New Jersey, Prentice-Hall, Inc., 1974.

California's Health, Vol. 29, No. 9, March, 1972 (special issue on venereal disease).

Cancer Facts and Figures, 1974, New York, American Cancer Society, Inc., 1974.

Cause of Death, Monthly Vital Statistics Report, Vol. 23, No. 3, Rockville, Md., U. S. Department of Health, Education, and Welfare, National Center for Health Statistics, May 24, 1974.

Chronic Conditions and Limitations of Activity and Mobility, Series 10, No. 61, Washington, D.C., U.S. Department of Health, Education, and Welfare, Public Health Service, 1971.

"Complexities of Gonococcal Infection," *Medical Aspects of Human Sexuality*, Vol. 6, No. 4, pp. 152–166, April 1972.

Conn, Howard F. (ed.), *Current Therapy 1974*, Philadelphia, W. B. Saunders Company, 1974.

Crouch, James E., *Functional Human Anatomy*, 2nd ed., Philadelphia, Lea & Febiger, 1972.

Frobisher, Martin and Robert Fuerst, *Microbiology in Health and Disease*, 13th ed., Philadelphia, W. B. Saunders Company, 1973.

"The Gonorrhea Epidemic and its Control," *Medical Aspects of Human Sexuality,* Vol. 5, No. 1, pp. 96–115, January 1971.

Guyton, Arthur C., *Textbook of Medical Physiology,* 4th ed., Philadelphia, W. B. Saunders Company, 1971.

Health in the Later Years of Life, Washington, D.C., U.S. Department of Health, Education, and Welfare, Public Health Service, 1971.

Jones, Kenneth L., Louis W. Shainberg, and Curtis O. Byer, *Dimensions,* 2nd ed., San Francisco, Canfield Press, 1974.

Jones, Kenneth L., Louis W. Shainberg, and Curtis O. Byer, *Health Science,* 3rd ed., New York, Harper & Row, Publishers, 1974.

Jones, Kenneth L., Louis W. Shainberg, and Curtis O. Byer, *VD,* New York, Harper & Row, Publishers, 1973.

Life Tables, Vital Statistics of the United States, 1971, Washington, D.C., U. S. Department of Health, Education, and Welfare, Public Health Service, 1974.

Mortality Trends: Age, Color, and Sex, Series 20, Number 15, Washington, D.C., U.S. Department of Health, Education, and Welfare, Public Health Service, 1973.

Prevalence of Selected Chronic Respiratory Conditions, Publication No. (HRA) 74–1511, Washington, D.C., U.S. Department of Health, Education, and Welfare, 1973.

Rheumatoid Arthritis in Adults, Series 11, Number 17, Washington, D.C., U.S. Department of Health, Education, and Welfare, Vital and Health Statistics, 1966.

Selye, Hans, *The Stress of Life,* New York, McGraw-Hill Book Company, 1956.

Smith, Alice Lorraine, *Microbiology and Pathology,* 10th ed., Saint Louis, The C. V. Mosby Company, 1972.

Smith, Alice Lorraine, *Principles of Microbiology,* 7th ed., Saint Louis, The C. V. Mosby Company, 1973.

Snively, W. D., Jr. and Donna R. Beshear, *Textbook of Pathophysiology,* Philadelphia, J. B. Lippincott Company, 1972.

Wilson, Marion E. and Helen Eckel Mizer, *Microbiology in Patient Care,* 2nd ed., New York, Macmillan Publishing Co., 1974.

INDEX

Italicized numbers indicate illustrations, charts, or tables. (Illustrations, charts, or tables occurring within a lengthy discussion are not singly identified unless they fall on the first or last page of the discussion.)

CP
3456789101112 75